WAISE KUR

Teaching and Learning Communication Skills in Medicine

Suzanne Kurtz
Jonathan Silverman
and
Juliet Draper

Forewords by

Barbara Korsch
Professor of Pediatrics
University of Southern California
School of Medicine

and

Sir David Weatherall
Regius Professor of Medicine
University of Oxford

Radcliffe Medical Press

Radcliffe Medical Press Ltd
18 Marcham Road, Abingdon, Oxon OX14 1AA, UK

British Library Cataloguing in Publication Data

A catalogue record for this book is available from the British Library.

ISBN 1 85775 273 2

Library of Congress Cataloging-in-Publication Data is available.

Typeset by Advance Typesetting Ltd, Oxon
Printed and bound by Bookcraft (Bath) Ltd

Contents

Foreword

These two texts on teaching and learning the skills of medical communication are a most welcome addition to the all too sparsely available literature on a topic which is now acknowledged to be crucial in the education and practice of all practitioners, and which is especially important for educators in the health professions. Together, these two books represent one more giant step forward in the evolution of our understanding of the patient–physician relationship and of communication skills in medicine.

What used to be considered the 'art' of medicine, a matter of intuition and personal attributes and hence unresearchable and certainly unteachable, has transmuted into a respectable field of science which is increasingly included explicitly in medical and related curricula. In spite of this evolution there has been a lack of data-based comprehensive literature on the subject. There is an impressive body of research and a large number of publications in the field of patient–clinician communication as such, but for the educator who needs to organize a curriculum, or even a single course, there has been little resource. Even though more institutions recognize the need for teaching this aspect of health care, there is a universal lack of trained faculty, and a deplorable lack of formalized credible documentation of sound principles for teaching this challenging subject. This lack makes it cumbersome for educators to formulate their teaching programme, as well as posing an additional barrier in the ever-continuing battle for a 'place in the sun', i.e. time in the curriculum to teach the doctor–patient relationship and related communication skills.

'What exactly is it that you want to teach?' is a question with which I have been challenged throughout my career. The text by Kurtz, Silverman and Draper contains the answer to this query. In a clear, concise but comprehensive manner the authors tell not only what, but also how and why communication skills should be learned and taught.

In this foreword there is no need to provide a detailed description of the two books' contents, the authors have done so very effectively in their introduction. I do want to underline one feature of the work that is of fundamental importance, namely that the material presented is carefully documented from available research. Data from the communication literature, including the important recent work relating not only outcomes such as patient satisfaction and compliance but also biological and functional patient outcomes to communication variables, are appropriately cited. In their presentation, the authors also bring together the growing body of evidence on the effectiveness of teaching about the doctor–patient relationship, and the duration of the desirable behaviour changes in the learner that can be achieved. Here again the authors provide valuable ammunition to the courageous proponents of teaching communication when challenged by their colleagues dealing with 'hard science' who consistently demand evidence for the value of this kind of teaching, even though the traditional aspects of medical education are frequently not submitted to this rigorous scrutiny.

The whole work is based on the principles for effective adult education. This is especially welcome because medical education, perhaps partly in light of the unfortunate tradition of considering the development of medical professionals as 'training' rather than education, is frequently not sufficiently learner-oriented. This in turn may contribute to clinicians' reluctance later in their practise to make their interactions sufficiently patient-centred. Thus this work, addressed to both learners and teachers, models the kind of communication that is being advocated.

Another welcome contribution is the emphasis on the integration and timing of communication teaching into the entire medical education programme instead of relegating the subject to one isolated course early in the curriculum, which may not even be a requirement, for which the students may not receive formal evaluation, which is considered a luxury not an essential, and which is the first to be cut when there is lack of time in the curriculum or when there is a fiscal exigency.

This work presents significant progress in the field of medical education at a time when there are dramatic changes in medical practice which make communication teaching mandatory and urgent.

Barbara Korsch
January 1998

Foreword

When these two extensive works on communication skills arrived on my desk I was reminded of that fine poem by John Dunne, *The Good Morrow,* in which he asks his lover whether there was any real existence before they met: 'Were we not weaned 'til then, But supped on country pleasures, childishly? Or snorted we in the seven sleepers' den?' As judged by recent attacks from all sides on its lack of ability to communicate, not to mention the rediscovery of 'evidence-based medicine', it appears that the medical profession has snorted happily for many centuries, or at least since the advent of high-technology practice and managed health care left it with neither the inclination nor time to sit down and talk to its patients.

While I suspect that at least a few physicians of the past must have been competent communicators, and it is only necessary to read of the life and work of Thomas Sydenham to realize that this must have been the case, it is certainly true that an awareness of the central role of fostering communication skills in medical education and clinical practice is a fairly recent phenomenon. During my time as a medical student in the 1950s, with the possible exception of developing a systemized approach to history taking, the subject was rarely mentioned. Rather, we were expected to learn how to interact with patients by osmosis, sitting dutifully hour after hour in outpatient departments watching the great men at work. I still vividly remember my first ward round with one of the most distinguished physicians in my teaching centre. We arrived at the bedside of a patient who had just been diagnosed as having carcinoma of the bronchus. We suddenly veered away from the bedside, formed a rugby scrum in the middle of the ward, whispered dire prognostications, returned briefly to the patient to utter a few meaningless banalities, and moved on. I have no idea who told that patient about the nature of his illness, if, indeed, anybody ever did. If bad news had to be broken, and so often it did, it was invariably left to the junior staff, who usually asked medical students to leave the room. I don't recall ever sitting in on a discussion about a terminal illness with a patient or their family. Overall, I suspect, we went out into the hard world totally unprepared for applying what is clearly the most important of all the clinical skills.

As will be plain to anybody who delves into these two excellent books, all this has changed. There is a growing awareness that communication is, together with an ability to listen, the most important aspect of practice that students and young (and not so young) doctors have to master. Modern high-technology diagnostic aids have not altered this fact. Indeed, with our increasingly ageing population and the extraordinarily complex ways in which diseases present and are forged by patients' lifestyles and environments, an ability to talk to our patients is becoming even more important. If the growing attractiveness of complementary medicine is telling us anything, it is that conventional western practice is losing its pastoral skills, particularly those which require both the time and ability to comfort sick people and their families.

Although it happens more often as one becomes a geriatric statistic, there is still no happier surprise and compliment than to be invited to write a foreword to a book by one of one's ex-students. In this case it is a particular pleasure because the subject is so important and central to many of the problems of the current clinical scene. What is even more encouraging to somebody who has tried, with limited success, to impress the importance of the scientific basis of medicine on young people is, as witnessed by these books, that considerable efforts are being made to try to measure the outcome of new approaches to teaching the skills of communication.

I hope that *all* those involved in medical education, and not a few students and doctors of all ages, will browse through these pages, lie in the bath and mull over what they have read, and then go straight to their wards, outpatients or practices and start really talking to sick people. While no amount of reading or teaching can make up for communicating directly with patients and their friends and families, and learning from one's mistakes over a lifetime, the modern approaches to improving this skill, so well presented in these books, are providing an increasingly valuable basis on which to build the most important of all the attributes that make for a good doctor.

David Weatherall
January 1998

Preface

Teaching and Learning Communication Skills in Medicine is one of two companion books which together provide a comprehensive approach to improving communication between doctors and patients throughout all three levels of medical education (undergraduate, residency and continuing medical education) and in both specialist and family medicine.

In this first book we examine how to construct a communication skills curriculum, document the individual skills that form the core content of communication skills teaching programmes and explore in depth the specific teaching and learning methods employed in this unique field of medical education. This book presents:

- an overall rationale for communication skills teaching – the 'why', the 'what' and the 'how' of teaching and learning communication skills in medicine
- the individual skills that constitute effective doctor–patient communication
- a systematic approach for presenting, learning and using these skills in practice
- a detailed description of appropriate teaching and learning methods, including:
  - innovative approaches to analysis and feedback in experiential teaching sessions
  - key facilitation skills that maximize participation and learning
- principles, concepts and research evidence that substantiate the specific teaching and learning methods used in communication skills programmes
- strategies for constructing a communication skills curriculum in practice.

In our second book, *Skills for Communicating with Patients*, we undertake a more detailed exploration of the specific skills of doctor–patient communication. We not only examine how to use these skills in the medical interview but also provide comprehensive evidence of the improvements that communication skills can make to both everyday clinical practice and to ensuing health outcomes. This second book presents:

- the individual skills that form the core content of communication skills teaching programmes
- an overall structure which helps organize the skills and our teaching and learning about them
- a detailed description and rationale for the use of each of these core skills in the medical interview

- principles, concepts and research evidence that validate the importance of the skills and document the potential gains for doctors and patients alike
- suggestions for how to use each skill in practice
- a discussion of the major role that these core communication skills play in tackling specific communication issues and challenges.

We encourage our readers to study both books. While at first glance it would appear that this book might be exclusively for teachers and its companion exclusively for learners, this is far from our intention:

- facilitators need as much help with 'what' to teach as 'how' to teach. We demonstrate how in-depth knowledge of the use of communication skills and of the accompanying research evidence is essential if facilitators wish to maximize learning in their experiential teaching sessions
- learners need to understand 'how' to learn as well as 'what' to learn. Understanding the principles of communication skills teaching will enable learners to maximize their own learning throughout the communication curriculum, improve their own participation in that learning, understand the value of observation and rehearsal, provide constructive feedback and contribute to the formation of a supportive climate.

In communication skills teaching there is a fine line between teachers and learners. Teachers will continue to make discoveries about communication throughout their professional lives and learn from their students. Learners not only teach their peers but soon become the communication skills teachers of the next generation of doctors, whether formally, informally or as role models. No doctor can escape this responsibility.

Suzanne Kurtz
Jonathan Silverman
Juliet Draper
January 1998

About this book

This book and its companion work are the result of a happy and fruitful collaboration between the three authors. It began with Dr Silverman taking a sabbatical with Professor Kurtz at the Faculty of Medicine, University of Calgary, Canada in 1993. Professor Kurtz and her colleagues have been developing and implementing communication curricula in medicine, as well as methods for improving communication in other areas of health care, since the mid 1970s. Dr Silverman and Dr Draper have been working together to run communication skills teaching in postgraduate general practice in the East Anglian region of the UK since 1989. Over the past four years the collaboration between the three authors has led to a cross-fertilization of ideas and methods and resulted in the writing of these two books.

Professor Kurtz and Dr Silverman share first authorship equally for both titles and to reflect this equality Professor Kurtz is listed as first author for *Teaching and Learning Communication Skills in Medicine* and Dr Silverman is listed as first author for *Skills for Communicating with Patients*.

About the authors

Dr Suzanne Kurtz, PhD, is Professor of Communication in the Faculties of Education and Medicine of the University of Calgary, Canada. Focusing her career on improving communication and educational practices in health care and education, development of communication curricula, and clinical skills evaluation, she has worked with medical and education students, residents, practising physicians, nurses, allied health professionals, patient groups, teachers and administrators. For over 20 years she has co-directed the undergraduate communication curriculum in Calgary's Faculty of Medicine and is called on nationally and internationally at all levels of medical education for her expertise in the specifics of setting up effective communication programmes. Working across diverse cultural and disciplinary lines, she has also collaborated on several international development projects related to health and education in Nepal, Southeast Asia, and Zululand. Her publications include an earlier book co-authored with VM Riccardi and entitled *Communication and counselling in health care* (Charles C Thomas, 1983).

Dr Jonathan Silverman, FRCGP, is a general practitioner in Linton, Cambridgeshire, and Communication Skills Teaching Facilitator for Postgraduate General Practice in the regional general practice office of the Anglia and Oxford Regional Health Authority. He has been a trainer for 10 years and was a course organizer of the Cambridge Vocational Training Scheme for five years. For the last eight years he has been organizer of the facilitator training programmes in general practice communication skills in East Anglia. In 1993, he was on sabbatical for six months, with the aid of BMA, RCGP and ACO travelling fellowships, working with Suzanne Kurtz, teaching and researching communication skills at the Faculty of Medicine, University of Calgary. He is at present developing a module in communication skills for the Masters Degree in Primary and Community Care at the University of Cambridge.

Dr Juliet Draper, FRCGP, MD, is a general practitioner in Cambridge and course organizer of the Cambridge Vocational Training Scheme. She is a trainer in general practice and organizer and evaluator of the facilitator training programmes in general practice communication skills in East Anglia. She has an MD in community antenatal care and has published on health visiting, consumer views on antenatal care and HRT. She has a particular interest in counselling in medical settings and has been involved in the development of the attachment of counsellors in primary care.

Acknowledgements

This book would not have been written without the help of patients, learners and colleagues from all over the world. They have taught us so much and we owe them a great debt.

Many people have helped us directly and indirectly with their ideas, support and time, in particular our families and the people we work with regularly – the preceptors and trainers in our courses, our partnerships and the secretaries, actors and audiovisual technicians who assist us.

We want especially to acknowledge Catherine Heaton, MD, for her creative work and continuous support over the past 15 years as co-director and co-author of the undergraduate communication curriculum in Calgary. Her substantive professional contributions to the teaching and evaluation programmes and her work with learners and patients have influenced our work and our books greatly.

We are particularly grateful to Bob Berrington and Arthur Hibble for providing protected time for us to write a manual for GP facilitators in the East Anglian region in 1996. This protected time provided a considerable impetus for the writing of this book. We also thank them for their continuing and enthusiastic support of communication training in East Anglia.

We are similarly grateful to Annette La Grange and Ian Winchester (Faculty of Education) and Penny Jennett, Al Jones, Henry Mandin, Eldon Smith and Wally Temple (Faculty of Medicine) for the sabbatical they made available to Professor Kurtz in 1996 to work on this book and for their ongoing and substantial administrative support of communication programmes at the University of Calgary.

For their advice, help and encouragement, we also sincerely thank Peter Campion, Arthur Clark, Brian Gromoff, David Haslam, Renee Martin, Tony Pearson, Meredith Simon and Sue Weaver.

Introduction

An evidence-based approach

The authors of this book believe passionately in the importance of communication skills in medicine; our overriding aim in writing this book is to help improve the standard of doctor–patient communication in practice. To achieve this aim, we have produced a practical text that enables facilitators, programme directors and learners at all levels of medical education to enhance their communication skills teaching and learning and that furthers the development of communication skills programmes. Improvements in education will lead directly to improvements in doctors' communication skills in practice which will, in turn, produce significant improvements in patient care and health outcomes.

Most previous texts have concentrated on communication in medicine *per se*; little has been written to help facilitators, programme directors and learners to come to terms with the practicalities of teaching and learning this subject. Yet our experience over many years is that communication skills teaching and learning, while highly rewarding, are complex and challenging tasks. This book therefore strives to:

- enhance the communication skills of *students, residents* and *established practitioners of medicine*
- enable *facilitators* and *learners* to move on from understanding the importance of communication to being able to teach and learn about it in practice
- provide *programme directors* and *facilitators* with the research evidence, concepts, principles and skills to teach this vital subject
- convince *medical educators* and *administrators* of the importance of developing excellent communication skills programmes within their institutions.

We also believe that there is a strong need to develop a unified and coherent approach to communication skills teaching. In this book we wish to:

- help coordinate the teaching of communication throughout the three levels of medical education, *undergraduate, residency* and *continuing medical education*
- demonstrate the importance of teaching and learning communication skills in *all specialties* of medicine and show the extensive common ground in both communication and communication skills teaching across all areas of clinical practice

- demonstrate just how similar the issues and challenges of communication skills teaching are across international boundaries and provide suggestions and solutions that are of equal value in *North America, Europe* and *other parts of the world*.

But belief and passion are not enough to produce changes in medical education. Without evidence to back our claims of subsequent widespread improvements in the practice of medicine, we cannot expect the relatively new discipline of communication to make substantial inroads into already crowded medical curricula. So our final aim of this book is to:

- provide an evidence-based approach to communication skills teaching and learning.

In this book we provide the concepts, principles and research evidence that validate the importance and efficacy of teaching and learning communication skills in medicine. In our companion volume, we explore in depth the individual skills of medical communication and document the considerable evidence that effective use of these skills can lead to improvements both in everyday clinical practice and in ensuing health outcomes for patients.

In this Introduction, we would like to explain the rationale behind our aims. We base our approach on the following premises.

Underlying premises

Communication is a core clinical skill essential to clinical competence

Knowledge, communication skills, problem solving and the physical examination are four essential components of clinical competence that together form the very essence of good clinical practice. Communication skills are not an optional extra in medical training: without appropriate communication skills, all our other clinical efforts can easily be wasted.

Communication is a learned skill that needs to be taught

Communication is not a personality trait but a series of learned skills. Communication in medicine needs to be taught with the same rigour as other core clinical skills, such as the physical examination.

Communication skills need to be taught effectively

Over the last two decades there has been increasing pressure from professional medical bodies to improve the training and evaluation of doctors in communication at both national (General Medical Council 1978; Association of American Medical Colleges 1984; American Board of Pediatrics 1987; Workshop Planning Committee 1992; Cowan and Laidlaw 1993; General Medical Council 1993; Barkun 1995; Royal College of Physicians 1997) and international levels (World Federation for Medical Education 1994). Yet, even where communication skills programmes have been adopted, they have not always been taught effectively (Novack *et al.*

1993; Whitehouse 1991). In this book, we examine the need to do more than just produce a programme that looks impressive on paper. Communication programmes need to produce effective and long-lasting changes in learners' communication skills. We examine the progress that has been made in establishing effective communication skills teaching in medicine, explore blocks to that progress and suggest ways to overcome these difficulties.

Communication skills teaching and learning is different

Communication skills teaching is different. It is not the same as teaching other subjects. Firstly, it has its own subject matter and methods. Knowing how to teach about cardiology does not necessarily equip you to teach communication skills. Knowing how to communicate in normal conversation is not the same as understanding the specific skills of communicating with patients. Communication in medicine is a professional skill that needs to be developed to a professional level. Secondly, learning communication is substantially different from learning cognitive content or other clinical skills. Communication skill is closely bound to self-concept, self-esteem and personality and this imposes added pressures on learners and facilitators. It is also much more complex than simpler procedural skills such as the physical examination. Learning interviewing is qualitatively and quantitatively different – while there is a ceiling in achievement for most skills (you can only get so good at them), this is not so for communication where the inherent complexity means that you can always learn more (Davidoff 1993). Thirdly, everyone comes with substantial experience and knowledge of communication – instead of starting from scratch as in, say, the physical examination, we all have some expertise. Fourthly, we have to work with our own and others' feelings in studying this subject, an aspect more easily avoided in more cognitive and technical areas of medical education.

Facilitators and programme directors need to know both the 'what' and the 'how' of communication skills teaching

Communication is a difficult subject to teach. The subject matter and methods are not necessarily well known among medical educators and teaching clinicians. Most communication facilitators and programme directors from a medical background were themselves educated in an era when communication skills were hardly taught at all. Too often it has been assumed that facilitators, through their very practice of medicine, will necessarily have gained sufficient knowledge of the specific skills involved in medical communication, the 'what' of communication skills teaching, and that all they need to learn is 'how' to teach this subject. This book, in contrast, places equal emphasis on educating facilitators and programme directors in the 'what' and the 'how'. Both are vitally important.

Communication skills teaching and learning needs to be evidence based

Comprehensive theoretical and research evidence now exists to guide our approach to communication skills teaching and learning. In this book, we demonstrate that certain teaching methods work in achieving long-lasting change in learners' behaviour. Twenty-five years of accumulated research also guides the choice of communication skills to include in the communication curriculum – we know which skills can actually make a difference in clinical practice. These research findings should now inform the education process and drive the communication skills curriculum forward (Stewart and Roter 1989, Simpson *et al.* 1991). In our companion volume, we provide this evidence in detail to help programme directors, facilitators and learners fully understand the underlying basis of the subject. Moreover, we present the evidence in a way that enables it to be actively used in the teaching process itself.

A unified approach to communication skills teaching in specialist and family medicine is needed

Some commentators have suggested that it is not possible for a text on communication skills teaching and learning to be appropriate to both general practice and the wide range of settings found in specialist medicine as these different contexts require very different skills. We disagree and feel strongly that these arguments have in the past been responsible for holding back the development of communication training. As many of the concepts and research efforts concerning communication skills were initially forged in general practice or psychiatry, it has been easy for specialists to say that the findings are irrelevant to the special needs of their work and that the lessons from one discipline cannot be transferred to another. The authors have considerable experience in teaching communication across a wide range of specialties and we have observed doctors' and medical students' communication skills in a wide variety of settings. While different contexts may require a subtle shift in emphasis, our overwhelming common experience is that the similarities far outweigh the differences and that the underlying principles and core communication skills remain the same: the barriers between specialties are more in subject matter than in communication skills. More recent research performed in secondary and tertiary care settings confirms our perceptions. In this book, we provide a coherent approach to teaching communication skills that highlights the core similarities yet still tackles the differences that occur in each context.

A unified approach to communication skills teaching which crosses cultural and national boundaries is possible

It has also been said that there are such important differences in culture, patient expectations, medical training, clinical management and health care systems between Britain, North America and other countries that it is very difficult to write a book on communication skills teaching which appeals to such a wide audience. Again, we disagree. The authors use the same techniques of teaching, the same principles of learning, and teach the same basic skills both in England and in Canada. Professor Kurtz in particular has observed medical consultations in many countries and cultures and has used identical methods to help develop communication programmes in medical settings in several developing countries. Undoubtedly, cultural differences which influence doctor–patient and teacher–learner relationships do exist and need to be taken into account; but in our experience, the similarities are far greater than the differences in both communication skills and communication skills teaching in all these different countries. Strangely, research and theory have not always travelled well between countries and teaching programmes tend not to take account of progress made elsewhere. The Toronto consensus statement (Simpson *et al.* 1991), multi-authored books such as Stewart and Roter's *Communication with medical patients* (1989) and international conferences have started to break down these international and cultural barriers. We would like to continue the process with this book.

A coordinated approach to communication skills teaching throughout undergraduate, residency and continuing medical education is necessary

We are especially keen to tie together the teaching of communication skills in undergraduate, residency and continuing medical education (CME). Again, we use the same methods of teaching, the same principles of learning and teach the same core skills in our work in undergraduate, residency and CME settings. This book demonstrates the need for a continuing, coherent programme of communication skills teaching that extends throughout all three levels of medical education, the need to both review and reiterate previous learning and the importance of moving on, deepening skills previously learned and adding new skills so as to meet more complex situations and challenges as learners advance from one level to the next. We show the need for a *coordinated curriculum* of communication skills teaching and how certain aspects of this are best dealt with at different times in learners' careers. We also discuss the different challenges to communication skills teaching at each of these three levels of education and consider how to work successfully in each environment. Again, we do not provide a book of rigid rules of how to teach but a flexible approach that allows facilitators to use and adapt available material and methods to suit their own specific circumstances.

A skill-based approach to communication skills teaching is essential

This book deliberately takes a predominantly skills-based approach to communication teaching rather than an attitude-based approach. Experiential skills-based teaching is the final common pathway that converts understanding, knowledge and attitudes into behaviour and action. Although we believe that it is important to tackle both skills and attitudes in communication programmes, we concentrate primarily in this book on the skills approach as it is the essential ingredient that enables change to occur in learners' behaviour. While cognitive or attitudinal work helps learners to understand the concepts of why we communicate in a certain way, only the skills approach provides the skills that enable learners to put these ideas and attitudes into practice.

Unlike many previously published texts, we also devote considerably more space to the teaching of core communication skills than the teaching of specific communication issues such as anger, addiction, ethics, multicultural and gender issues. Core skills are fundamental: once they have been mastered, more specific communication issues and challenges are much more readily tackled. To our mind, other medical communication texts have moved on to specific issues too quickly without devoting enough time to more fundamental skills. Our approach is therefore to expend more effort on core skills than issues. Although we feel that specific communication issues are highly important and must be included in communication programmes, such issues should not be presented as if each is a completely new problem unrelated to core skills. Instead, issues should be used to demonstrate how core skills can be employed in specific circumstances and what additional issue-specific skills need to be superimposed upon them. In this book, we explore how to teach about skills, attitudes and issues in a predominantly skills-based programme.

Who are the intended audience for this book?

Facilitators and programme directors

One major audience for this book are the facilitators and programme directors involved in teaching, planning and developing communication skills programmes, whether in undergraduate, residency or continuing medical education, in specialist training or general practice, or in North America, Europe or other parts of the world. We recognize that these readers are not a uniform group and may come from the following very diverse backgrounds:

- medical
  - community, hospital or academic-based doctors
  - general practice and family practice physicians
  - psychiatrists
  - specialists
  - nurses
  - allied health professionals
- non-medical
  - communication specialists
  - psychology or counselling backgrounds.

This diversity has caused some stylistic difficulties in writing this book. Often in the book we have chosen to refer to facilitators as if they are all doctors – we might quote the facilitator as saying to a learner group 'We all have similar problems with patients' even though our readers, like the three authors of this book, are not all medical practitioners. We use this device because we feel it is preferable to saying 'What you doctors all do is…'. It is helpful to include ourselves in such descriptions, even if we are not all doctors, so as to align ourselves with the medical profession rather than being seen to be 'doctor bashing'. Those of us who are not doctors have interactions with our learners that are similar to the interactions doctors have with their patients and the lessons are very similar for us all. Hopefully, non-medical facilitators will also understand that we are not implying that all facilitators are, or should be, doctors.

Learners at all levels of medical education

We are keen for learners to read this book as well as its companion volume which discusses the 'what' of communication skills programmes in greater depth. Understanding the 'how' of communication skills teaching and learning will enable learners to improve their own participation by understanding the point of observation, the need for contributing to a supportive climate and the importance of constructive feedback from all members of the group. In communication skills programmes, learners become significant 'facilitators' of each other's learning. In addition, all doctors need to understand principles of education and change even if they are not intending to be medical educators: doctors are all involved in educating patients even if they do not educate other doctors.

Residents and practising doctors

Whether as learners themselves, informal teachers in the workplace or role models to the next generation of doctors, it is important for practising doctors and residents to understand communication skills and communication skills teaching.

Medical education administrators, funding agencies and medical politicians

It is vital for those in positions of authority and power to understand the importance of communication skills teaching and learning. It is also vital that deans of medical institutions, administrators of health management organizations (HMOs), hospitals and health authorities, medical societies, royal colleges, medical associations, funding agencies and politicians appreciate the resources, manpower and curriculum time required to develop and sustain a successful communication programme.

Organization of the book

To make access to this resource easier for such a diverse audience, we have divided the book into three interrelated parts:

- **Part 1** presents an overview of the 'why', 'what' and 'how' of teaching and learning communication skills in medicine – the core of communication curricula
- **Part 2** explores how to pull these elements together and apply them in practice. Whether you are just becoming involved in this area or looking for alternatives to improve your current practice, this section offers strategies, skills and insights for teaching and learning communication in medicine. Many of these resources also apply to working more effectively with patients
- **Part 3** examines the issues and challenges surrounding the development of communication curricula in medicine and anticipates directions for communication curricula of the future.

This book is designed to be used both as a complete package and as a handbook which can be dipped into as need and interest dictate.

How have we addressed style issues in a book intended for both a European and North American market?

A particular problem of this book has been how to write for a diverse audience. So many words and phrases have subtly different meanings that we have had to tread carefully to avoid unnecessary confusion. Throughout the book, we have decided to use certain words consistently; we apologise for this shorthand and hope that readers will be able to translate our convention to fit their own context. For instance, we have tried to use:

specialist rather than *consultant*
resident rather than *registrar* or *trainee*
programme director rather than *course organizer*
facilitator rather than *preceptor, trainer* or *tutor*
learner rather than *student*
office rather than *surgery*
follow-up interview rather than *review*
continuing medical education (CME) rather than *continuing professional education (CPD).*

Some areas have proved to be more difficult. We use *medical interview* and *consultation* interchangeably. We also use the British *general practice* and North American *family medicine* to mean the same, despite their different meanings in North America.

Part 1

An overview of communication skills teaching and learning

1

The 'why': a rationale for communication skills teaching and learning

Introduction

Let us start at the beginning – why embark on trying to teach communication skills at all? Why do we feel it is so important? What justification is there for expending the effort in an already overcrowded timetable for learning? Why should curriculum organizers at all three levels of medical education – undergraduate, residency and continuing medical education – adopt this relatively new subject with enthusiasm and organize communication skills teaching within their own programmes? And if they do, will it work? Will it produce effective and long-lasting change in learners' communication skills or simply look impressive on paper? Is it just a sop to the authorities to allow your institution to say 'We're doing something – see'? Or is it sufficiently grounded in theory and research to enable you to say 'All this effort is worth it – our learners and their patients will truly benefit, both now and in the future'?

In this chapter we provide a rationale for communication skills teaching that is based squarely on theory and research. To do that, we must answer the following questions:

- Why teach and learn communication skills?
  - is it important to study the medical interview?
  - are there problems in communication between doctors and patients?
  - is there evidence that communication skills can overcome these problems and make a difference to patients, doctors and outcomes of care?
- Can you teach and learn communication skills?
  - is there evidence that communication skills can be taught and learned?
  - is there evidence that learning is retained?

- Is the prize on offer to doctors and patients worth the effort?
  - will expending the effort on communication skills teaching produce worthwhile rewards for both doctors and patients?

If the answer to any of these questions is 'no' then we can all relax and get back to our programmes without worrying about yet another change. But if the answer to these questions is 'yes' then our work is cut out for the future and we ignore communication skills teaching at our peril.

Why teach communication skills?

Is it important to study the medical interview?

- The medical interview is central to clinical practice. It has been estimated that doctors perform 200 000 consultations in a professional lifetime so it is worth struggling to get it right.
- The interview is *the* unit of medical time, a critical few minutes for the doctor to help the patient with their problems. While the doctor may see each consultation as one of many routine encounters, for the patient it may be the most important or stressful aspect of their week.
- To achieve an effective interview, doctors need to be able to integrate four aspects of their work which together determine their overall clinical competence:
  - knowledge
  - communication skills
  - problem solving
  - physical examination.
- These four essential components of clinical competence are inextricably linked: outstanding expertise in any one alone is not sufficient. It is, for example, not good enough to be factually excellent if communication difficulties stand between you and the patient and prevent you from discovering the reason for the patient's attendance or from discussing a plan that the patient can understand and wishes to put into action. Communication is a core clinical skill rather than an optional extra.
- How we communicate is just as important as what we say. Communication bridges the gap between evidence-based medicine and working with individual patients.

Are there problems in communication between doctors and patients?

In our companion book we describe in detail the research evidence which demonstrates that there are substantial problems in communication between doctors and patients. Here we simply provide examples of this research to spur your interest to delve deeper into our companion volume.

DISCOVERING THE REASONS FOR THE PATIENT'S ATTENDANCE

- Fifty-four per cent of patients' complaints and 45% of their concerns are not elicited (Stewart *et al.* 1979).
- In 50% of visits, the patient and the doctor do not agree on the nature of the main presenting problem (Starfield *et al.* 1981).
- Doctors frequently interrupt patients so soon after they begin their opening statement that patients fail to disclose significant concerns (Beckman and Frankel 1984).
- Doctors often interrupt patients after the initial concern, apparently assuming that the first complaint is the chief one, yet the order in which patients present their problems is not related to their clinical importance (Beckman and Frankel 1984).

GATHERING INFORMATION

- Doctors often pursue a 'doctor-centred', closed approach to information gathering that discourages patients from telling their story or voicing their concerns (Byrne and Long 1976).
- Both a 'high control style.' and premature focus on medical problems can lead to an overnarrow approach to hypothesis generation and to inaccurate consultations (Platt and McMath 1979).
- Doctors rarely ask their patients to volunteer their ideas and, in fact, doctors often evade their patients' ideas and inhibit their expression. Yet if discordance between doctors' and patients' ideas and beliefs about the illness remains unrecognized, poor understanding, adherence, satisfaction and outcome are likely to ensue (Tuckett *et al.* 1985).

EXPLANATION AND PLANNING

- In general, physicians give sparse information to their patients, with most patients wanting their doctors to provide more information than they do (Waitzkin 1984; Beisecker and Beisecker 1990; Pinder 1990).
- Doctors overestimate the time they devote to explanation and planning in the consultation by up to 900% (Waitzkin 1984; Makoul *et al.* 1995).
- Patients and doctors disagree over the relative importance of imparting different types of medical information: patients place the highest value on information about prognosis, diagnosis and causation of their condition while doctors overestimate their patients' desire for information concerning treatment and drug therapy (Kindelan and Kent 1987).
- Doctors consistently use jargon that patients do not understand (Svarstad 1974; Hadlow and Pitts 1991).
- There are significant problems with patients' recall and understanding of the information that doctors impart (Tuckett *et al.* 1985).

PATIENT ADHERENCE

- Patients do not comply or adhere to the plans that doctors make: on average, 50% do not take their medicine at all or take it incorrectly (Meichenbaum and Turk 1987; Butler *et al.* 1996).
- Non-compliance is enormously expensive. In 1980, Walton *et al.* estimated that the cost of such wasted drugs per year in the UK was in the order of £300 million; more recent estimates

of the overall costs of non-compliance (including extra visits to physicians, laboratory tests, additional medications, hospital and nursing home admissions, lost productivity and premature death) are CAN\$7–9 billion in Canada (Coambs *et al.* 1995) and US\$100 billion plus in the United States (Berg *et al.* 1993).

MEDICO-LEGAL ISSUES

- Breakdown in communication between patients and physicians is a critical factor leading to malpractice litigation (Levinson 1994). Lawyers identified physicians' communication and attitudes as the primary reason for patients pursuing a malpractice suit in 70% of cases (Avery 1986). Beckman *et al.* (1994) showed that the following four communication problems were present in over 70% of malpractice depositions: deserting the patient, devaluing patients' views, delivering information poorly and failing to understand patients' perspectives.
- In several states of the USA, malpractice insurance companies award premium discounts of 3–10% annually to their insured physicians who attend a communication skills workshop (Carroll 1996).

LACK OF EMPATHY AND UNDERSTANDING

- Numerous reports of patient dissatisfaction with the doctor–patient relationship appear in the media. Many articles comment on doctors' lack of understanding of the patient as a person with individual concerns and wishes.
- In medical education significant problems exist in the development of relationship-building skills; it is not correct to assume that doctors either have the ability to communicate empathically with their patients or that they will acquire this ability during their medical training (Sanson-Fisher and Poole 1978).

Is there evidence that communication skills can overcome these problems and make a difference to patients, doctors and outcomes of care?

So there are plenty of problems, but are there solutions? In our companion volume we document in detail the evidence that the use of specific communication skills can overcome the very problems that we have listed above. Although here again we provide only a few examples to whet your appetite, many studies over the last 25 years have demonstrated that communication skills can make a difference in all of the following objective measurements of medical care.

PROCESS OF THE INTERVIEW

- The longer the doctor waits before interrupting at the beginning of the interview, the more likely she is to discover the full spread of issues that the patient wants to discuss and the less likely will it be that new complaints arise at the end of the interview (Beckman and Frankel 1984; Joos *et al.* 1996).

- The use of open rather than closed questions and the use of attentive listening leads to greater disclosure of patients' significant concerns (Cox 1989; Wissow *et al.* 1994; Maguire *et al.* 1996).
- Asking 'What worries you about this problem?' is not as effective a question as 'What concerns you about this problem?' in discovering unrecognized concerns (Bass and Cohen 1982).
- The more questions patients are allowed to ask of the doctor, the more information they obtain (Tuckett *et al.* 1985).

PATIENT SATISFACTION

- Greater 'patient centredness' in the interview leads to greater patient satisfaction (Stewart 1984; Arborelius and Bremberg 1992).
- Discovering and acknowledging patients' expectations improves patient satisfaction (Korsch *et al.* 1968; Eisenthal and Lazare 1976; Eisenthal *et al.* 1990).
- Physician non-verbal communication (eye contact, posture, nods, appropriate distance, communication of emotion though face and voice) is positively related to patient satisfaction (Larsen and Smith 1981; Weinberger *et al.* 1981; DiMatteo *et al.* 1986).
- Patient satisfaction is directly related to the amount of information that patients perceive they have been given by their doctors (Hall *et al.* 1988).

PATIENT RECALL AND UNDERSTANDING

- Asking patients to repeat in their own words what they understand of the information they have just been given increases their retention of that information by 30% (Bertakis 1977).
- There is decreased understanding of information given if the patient's and doctor's explanatory frameworks are at odds and if this is not discovered and addressed during the interview (Tuckett *et al.* 1985).
- Patient recall is increased by categorization, signposting, summarizing, repetition, clarity and use of diagrams (Ley 1988).

ADHERENCE

- Patients who are viewed as partners, informed of treatment rationales and helped in understanding their disease are more adherent to plans made (Schulman 1979).
- Doctors can increase adherence to treatment regimens by explicitly asking patients about knowledge, beliefs, concerns and attitudes to their own illness (Inui *et al.* 1976; Maiman *et al.* 1988).
- Discovering patients' expectations leads to greater patient adherence to plans made whether or not those expectations are met by the doctor (Eisenthal and Lazare 1976; Eisenthal *et al.* 1990).

OUTCOME

Symptom resolution:
- Resolution of symptoms of chronic headache is more related to the patient's feeling that they were able to discuss their headache and problems fully at the initial visit with their

doctor than to diagnosis, investigation, prescription or referral (The Headache Study Group 1986).

- Training doctors in problem-defining and emotion-handling skills not only leads to improvements in the detection of psychosocial problems but also to a reduction in patients' emotional distress up to six months later (Roter *et al.* 1995).

Physiological outcome:

- Giving the patient the opportunity to discuss their health concerns rather than simply answer closed questions leads to better control of hypertension (Orth *et al.* 1987).
- Decreased need for analgesia after myocardial infarction is related to information giving and discussion with the patient (Mumford *et al.* 1982).
- Providing an atmosphere in which the patient can be involved in choices if they are available leads to less anxiety and depression after breast cancer surgery (Fallowfield *et al.* 1990).
- Patients who are coached in asking questions of, and negotiating with, their doctor not only obtain more information but actually achieve better blood pressure control in hypertension and improved blood sugar control in diabetes (Kaplan *et al.* 1989; Rost *et al.* 1991).

Can you teach and learn communication skills?

So, problems exist in doctor–patient communication and specific communication skills can provide solutions. But can these communication skills be taught? Isn't it all a matter of learning by experience or osmosis? Surely you cannot short cut the learning that occurs through having to deal with many difficult situations over a professional lifetime? Maybe we learn best just by watching our superiors do it. Anyway, isn't it really a matter of personality, that some people can do it and others will never be able to? Isn't trying to define what makes for good communication and breaking it down into its constituent parts a bit like trying to understand what makes one actor have stage presence and the other seem wooden? You can teach each little bit but the sum of the parts does not add up to the whole – so why bother?

All these questions are genuine comments from participants at the beginning of our own communication courses and demand answers. If they are correct in their implications and communication skills are not teachable, we can abandon our efforts and save ourselves a lot of effort right now. What then is our rationale for thinking that communication skills can and should be taught?

- Communication is a core clinical skill.
- It is a series of learned skills.
- Experience can be a poor teacher of communication skills.
- Communication can be taught.
- Changes resulting from communication skills training can be retained.
- Specific learning methods are required to obtain change.

Communication is a clinical skill

Effective communication between patient and doctor is a basic clinical skill which demands teaching just as much as the physical examination. It is increasingly recognized that it can and should be taught with the same rigour as other basic medical sciences. We would not dream of omitting the teaching of the physical examination: we carefully observe learners' performance both in practice and in evaluations. Yet we do not take the same interest in how learners communicate with patients, despite the fact that history taking is known to contribute more to making a diagnosis than the examination (Hampton *et al.* 1975; Peterson *et al.* 1992).

It is a series of learned skills

Communication in medicine is a *series* of *learned* skills rather than just a matter of personality. Of course, personality is important but much of our ability to communicate has been learned and is not simply inherent in our genetic make-up. While we may have been born with a predisposition to communicate and interact with others, how well we develop these characteristics is strongly influenced by what we learn from our environment, experience and education.

Personality may well provide a head start but we can all learn from wherever our individual starting point may be. Some have a predisposition to play golf, a natural eye–hand coordination which places them at an advantage over others. But this does not mean that someone without this inbuilt ability cannot improve their golf by learning to be more skilled or that the expert golfer does not require constant attention to his skills so that he can improve even more. Anyone who wants to can learn.

The key to learning a complicated skill, be it a sport or communicating with patients, is to break the composite skill into its constituent parts. We often say 'She's good with patients' or 'She really has a nice style, it all seemed so easy' without quite identifying what she did, thereby making it difficult to emulate. We need instead to identify the actual skills that have been used, practise the individual components and then put them back together again into a seamless whole. You would not expect to learn tennis by watching a grand-slam match and saying 'Now that I've seen great tennis, I'll play some'! We need to identify the *series* of skills that make up the whole, and this has to be at quite a detailed level. Our tennis coach just telling us how to do a good forehand drive is also not enough: we may not be holding the racquet at the appropriate angle or standing in an optimal position and will never know if these individual skill components are not identified through coaching.

Experience can be a poor teacher

Unfortunately, communication skills do not necessarily improve with time and experience may well be a poor teacher. We know from the work of Byrne and Long (1976) and Ridsdale *et al.* (1992) that doctors tend to adopt a set, unvarying style of consulting which they use for all patients repeatedly and consistently, and that there appears to be no relationship between either the doctor's age or time available in the consultation and the use of specific interviewing skills. Sadly, experience may be simply an excellent reinforcer of bad habits: despite obvious deficiencies in consulting technique that are counterproductive to even basic doctor–patient communication, doctors persistently use the same methods over and over again. We become fixed in a rut. And our own perception of what we do as communicators is not necessarily accurate; for example, Waitzkin (1984) found that doctors devoted little more than one minute on average to the task of information giving in interviews lasting 20 minutes but overestimated the amount of time they spent on this task by a factor of nine.

We also know that without specific training in communication skills, medical students' ability to communicate tends to deteriorate as they progress through their traditional medical training. They enter medical school with better communicating skills than when they leave. The actual process of medical training, of adopting the medical model and thought processes, decreases their ability to communicate with patients.

Helfer (1970) showed that medical students' communication skills got worse as they proceeded through their training. As students moved through training, their ability to communicate with mothers of ill children was diminished by their increasing desire to obtain factual information. Traditional methods of medical education erode medical students' interpersonal and interviewing skills (Association of American Medical Colleges 1984).

Maguire and Rutter (1976) showed serious deficiencies in senior medical students' information-gathering skills without specific training: few students managed to discover the patient's main problem, clarify the exact nature of the problem, explore ambiguous statements, clarify with precision, elicit the impact of the problem on daily life, respond to verbal cues, cover more personal topics or use facilitation. Most used closed, lengthy, multiple and repetitive questions. Irwin and Bamber (1984) found similar deficiencies in key interviewing skills: they found problems with clarification, silence, confronting, picking up non-verbal leads and in covering psychological, personal and social aspects.

Maguire, Fairbairn and Fletcher (1986b) looked at the information-giving skills of two groups of young doctors, one group who five years previously had completed feedback training in information gathering at medical school and another group who had not received the benefit of this experience. The interview skills training given had, however, not included any formal training in information giving *per se*. The results were disturbing. In both groups doctors were weakest in those very information-giving techniques that have been found to increase patients' satisfaction and compliance with advice and treatment. Although there were clear differences in information-gathering skills between those who had completed the course on interviewing skills at medical school and those who had been controls, no difference at all in information-giving skills was detected. This demonstrates that doctors cannot rely on experience alone to be their guide and that they need specific communication training in each section of the interview if they wish to become effective throughout the consultation.

More recently, Davis and Nicholaou (1992) have shown improvements in interviewing skills as students progress through medical school: they surmise that this change from previous findings may relate to alterations in approaches and attitudes to communication training over the last two decades.

Specific communication skills teaching does produce change in learners' skills: interview skills can be taught

For over 20 years we have had clear evidence that specific communication skills training can lead to improvements in doctors' communication skills: that interview skills can be taught is now beyond doubt.

Rutter and Maguire (1976) showed in a controlled trial that medical students who underwent a training programme in history-taking skills during their psychiatry clerkship reported almost three times as much relevant and accurate information after a test interview as those who received only the traditional apprenticeship method of learning history-taking skills.

These immediate effects of training medical students have been confirmed by Irwin and Bamber (1984) and Evans *et al.* (1989). Evans *et al.* (1991) have also shown that medical students who learned key interviewing skills were diagnostically more efficient and effective in interviewing medical and surgical patients (i.e. that the improved behaviours and skills developed in training led to an increase in clinical proficiency) and yet took no more time with interviews than untrained students.

Similar findings have been replicated in many different settings:

- Stillman *et al.* (1976, 1977) showed the effectiveness of using simulated patients in improving medical students' interviewing skills in their paediatric clerkship.
- Sanson-Fisher and Poole (1978) showed the effectiveness of training undergraduate medical students in empathy skills.
- Putnam *et al.* (1988) and Joos *et al.* (1996) showed that training internal medical residents and staff physicians to use more appropriate interviewing skills led to significant improvements in the information-gathering process.
- Goldberg *et al.* (1980) showed that similar interview training could increase the accuracy with which family doctors were able to recognize psychiatric illness.
- Gask *et al.* (1987, 1988) showed that the interviewing skills of both trainers and registrars in family practice can be improved by communication skills training.
- Levinson and Roter (1993) showed potentially important changes in practising family physicians after a three-day continuing medical education (CME) programme.
- Inui *et al.* (1976) looked at the effect of a single training session on compliance-aiding interviewing skills given to physicians working with patients with known hypertension in out-patient clinics. Trained doctors spent more time in considering their patients' ideas and in patient education than did control physicians, patients' understanding of their condition improved and compliance increased. Most startlingly, however, there was also better control of hypertension even six months after the tutorial!
- Roter *et al.* (1995) showed in a randomized controlled trial that an eight-hour communication skills course in CME for primary care physicians not only improved the detection and management of psychosocial problems but also led to reduction in patients' emotional distress.

In Chapter 3, we explore the teaching methods that were used in these studies to bring about such impressive changes in learners' communication skills.

The changes resulting from communication skills training can be retained

Gratifyingly, more than just short-term gains have been demonstrated. Changes in learners' communication skills have been shown to be long-lasting:

- Maguire *et al.* (1986a) followed up their original students five years after their training. They found that both groups had improved but those given communication skills training had maintained their superiority in key skills such as using open questions, clarification, picking up verbal cues and coverage of psychosocial issues. These effects were found in interviews with patients with both psychiatric and physical illnesses.

- Stillman *et al.* (1977) demonstrated that trained students maintained their post-training superiority over their non-trained peers at follow-up a year later.
- Bowman *et al.* (1992) showed that the improvement in interviewing skills of established general practitioners following an interview training course, as described in Gask *et al.* (1987), was maintained over a two-year follow-up period.

Specific learning methods are required to obtain change

In Chapter 3 we explore in greater depth the evidence that certain experiential methods of learning are required to enable learners to change their behaviour in the consultation. We shall see how the studies above clearly point us in the direction of:

- systematic delineation and definition of essential skills
- observation
- well-intentioned, detailed and descriptive feedback
- video or audio recording and review
- practice and rehearsal of skills
- active small group or one-to-one learning

and that, by themselves, neither traditional apprenticeship nor didactic teaching methods will achieve change in specific behaviours or skills.

Is the prize on offer to doctors and patients worth the effort?

What then does communication skills training offer to doctors and their patients? Communication is not, as some would say, simply good manners, being nice or 'pandering to the patient'. The prize on offer is much greater than this: communication skills training promises more effective consultations and improved outcomes for both patients and doctors.

More effective consultations

In the discussion above we have seen that communication skills can produce more effective consultations for both patients and doctors. However knowledgeable doctors are about the facts of medicine, without appropriate communication skills they may not be able to:

- efficiently discover the problems or issues that the patient wishes to address
- accurately obtain the full history
- jointly make an acceptable, understood management plan that patients can adhere to
- supportively form a relationship that helps reduce conflicts for both patient and doctor.

The appropriate use of communication skills enables doctors to accomplish three goals that are essential to the effectiveness of every consultation (Riccardi and Kurtz 1983):

1 accuracy
2 efficiency
3 supportiveness.

Improved outcomes

We have also seen how communication can significantly improve health outcomes for patients: individual skills can lead to improvements in patient satisfaction, adherence, symptom relief and physiological outcome. Effective communication makes a difference to patients' health.

Communication can also improve outcomes for doctors. The use of appropriate communication skills not only increases patients' satisfaction with their doctors but also helps doctors to feel less frustrated and more satisfied in their work (Levinson *et al.* 1993). Appropriate communication reduces conflict by preventing the misunderstanding which is so often the source of difficulties between doctors and patients.

What can we say to our institutions to convince them of the need to run communication skills programmes?

The message to our institutions is not just that we can provide a more patient-centred approach to the interview. However laudable an aim that is, however important we might see the need to discover patients' concerns and needs and to involve patients more in the consultation, it often cuts little ice with those who have yet to see the light. The really important selling point is simple: *effective communication is essential to the practice of high-quality medicine*. By establishing communication skills programmes we can enable learners to improve their clinical performance. They will be more accurate and efficient diagnosticians and they will have patients who both understand and adhere to proposed management plans. Ultimately, learners will enhance their ability to work with patients – to improve health, manage illness and even achieve better physiological outcomes.

2

The 'what': defining what exactly we are trying to teach and learn

Introduction

So far we have seen that:

- teaching and learning about medical communication is important
- there are definite problems in doctor–patient communication
- there are proven solutions to these problems
- communication skills can be taught and learned
- communication skills teaching can be retained.

But is it clear what exactly we are trying to teach and learn? Can we define the individual skills of medical communication? Is it possible to break down such a complex and important task as the consultation into its individual components?

In our communication skills courses, learners at all levels often start by saying: 'Isn't it all subjective? Where is the evidence to validate what you are saying? What is the curriculum of communication skills – it all seems to be just a disorganized bag of tricks. How much breadth is there to this subject – I know one or two skills to focus on but perhaps I'm missing out whole chunks that I'm just not aware of?' These questions all deserve answers. To teach and learn communication skills we must be able to define the individual skills that make a difference to medical communication. We need to validate these skills by presenting the theoretical and research evidence that justifies their inclusion in our communication programmes; and we must generate a conceptual framework that enables learners and facilitators to make sense of both the individual skills and how they relate to the consultation as a whole.

In this chapter we therefore:

- explore why facilitators and programme directors may need help with knowing what to teach about communication skills
- define the broad types of skills that constitute doctor–patient communication
- describe a curriculum of skills in the form of the *Calgary–Cambridge observation guide*
- describe a framework for organizing the skills and explain why this structure is important
- discuss the theoretical and research basis for choosing the skills to include in the communication curriculum.

Why facilitators and programme directors need help with knowing what to teach

If one aim of this book is to help facilitators and programme directors teach communication skills in medicine, why do we place equal emphasis on both 'what' and 'how' to teach and learn communication skills? Can we not just omit the 'what' and move straight to the 'how'? Surely non-medical facilitators will have a background in communication studies and know the 'what' already. And won't medically trained facilitators also know the subject matter of communication skills programmes – after all, they use these skills every day in their clinical practice? Surely knowing what to teach is easy, it's discovering the correct teaching methodology that's difficult, especially for doctors who for the most part have had little previous training in teaching methods.

Over the years we have discovered that these are potentially dangerous assumptions. We have come to realize that facilitator training programmes, and hence this book, need to concentrate equally on the 'what' and the 'how' of communication skills teaching. Teachers who feel at ease with the range of teaching methods and their ability to run sessions often still feel uncomfortable with the subject matter itself. The following are typical of comments heard even from our experienced facilitators: 'I just can't figure out what to focus on'; 'I seem to just teach on a few bits and pieces here and there'; 'My feedback seems too random'; 'I'm not sure if I picked up on all the right things to teach'; 'I'm not sure if what I teach has any validity or is just my own ideas'. Not surprisingly, facilitators' difficulties with content and structure are often mirrored in the experience of their learners. But where does this difficulty with content come from?

- Most doctors who become communication skills facilitators received little communication training themselves during their own education. In fact, there may have been no teaching at all of communication skills when they were at medical school. Their own 'communication training' has frequently been gained entirely from their experience as doctors. Unfortunately, as we have seen in Chapter 1, experience alone is generally an insufficient training in this area, often serving only as an excellent reinforcer of bad habits (Helfer 1970; Byrne and Long 1976; Maguire *et al.* 1986a). So doctors may not have acquired the knowledge base or received the benefit of formal communication training themselves. Although they may be highly interested, facilitators may well not be fully comfortable or practised in the skills that they are trying to teach.

- Many non-medical facilitators come from allied fields such as psychology and counselling – like doctors, they may have had little formal training in communication. Even those from a communication background may not have studied doctor–patient communication *per se*.
- Considerable evidence has accumulated over the last 25 years that enables us to define the skills that enhance communication between patient and physician and that can be promoted as behaviours worth teaching and learning. However, both medical and non-medical facilitators have found it difficult to access the literature as it appears in such a wide variety of specialist journals and many facilitators have only limited time to keep up to date with the research. As a result, this information has not been widely disseminated and facilitators often feel uncertain of the validity of their teaching. This is a particular difficulty in communication training where small-group or one-to-one teaching necessitates the involvement of a large number of facilitators, all of whom need to be able to understand this evidence and use it in their teaching.
- Facilitators often do not have a clear conceptual framework to enable them to think systematically about communication in the medical interview and within which to pull together and organize the specific skills that they identify as worth learning. Consequently, the numerous skills often appear to be just a disorganized bag of tricks. Facilitators have problems piecing the individual skills together to ensure systematic development and understanding of communication skills.

The blind leading the blind

We cannot assume that facilitators necessarily have a better grasp of the subject matter than their learners. Facilitators may never have been taught communication formally and may not necessarily demonstrate high standards of communication in their own practice. Even if they are good communicators, they may have never analysed what they do and so may have difficulty in teaching it. This situation has been described as the blind leading the blind or even nowadays, at postgraduate level, the blind leading the partially sighted, as increasingly, medical students and more recently trained doctors have had more training in this subject than those attempting to teach them!

Helping facilitators to understand the 'what' of communication skills teaching is beneficial in several ways. Firstly, because many medical facilitators have been denied any significant communication skills training in their own previous education, it is important for them to have an opportunity to address their own communication skills and extend their own personal understanding of the 'what' of communication training. Secondly, understanding the 'what' will help them immeasurably in their teaching. To teach well, it is important for facilitators to develop an excellent grasp of the skills that are worth teaching, the research and theoretical evidence that validates the use of specific communication skills, the overall breadth of the communication skills curriculum and a conceptual framework or structure within which to organize the skills. It is easy otherwise to be random in our teaching, to forget key communication skills or even neglect whole chunks of the interview such as explanation and planning.

We are especially keen that facilitators understand the research evidence underlying communication skills and become adept at using this knowledge in their teaching. A particular feature of good experiential communication skills teaching is the ability of the facilitator to introduce cognitive material or research evidence at just the point in the learners' experiential deliberations when they have generated a need for information and when it will therefore be most readily assimilated. The facilitator is not simply guiding a self-directed learning group but has expertise and information that, if sensitively introduced, can greatly illuminate experiential learning.

Defining the broad types of communication skills

What are we actually studying in communication programmes? We begin our answer to this question by defining three types of communication skills that need to be addressed in communication skills curricula:

1 **Content skills.** What doctors communicate – the substance of their questions and responses; the information they gather and give; the treatments they discuss
2 **Process skills.** How they do it – the ways they communicate with patients; how they go about discovering the history or providing information; the verbal and non-verbal skills they use; how they develop the relationship with the patient; the way they organize and structure communication
3 **Perceptual skills.** What they are thinking and feeling – their internal decision making, clinical reasoning and problem solving; their awareness of feelings and thoughts about the patient, about the illness and about other issues that may be concerning them; awareness of their own self-concept and confidence, of their own biases, attitudes, intentions and distractions.

It is important to emphasize that content, process and perceptual skills are inextricably linked and cannot be considered in isolation. We must give attention to all three types when studying the medical interview (Riccardi and Kurtz 1983; Beckman and Frankel 1994).

Below are some examples which demonstrate this interdependence.

EXAMPLE 1
Say you ask a series of closed questions (process) early on in the consultation about one specific area (content). This apparently efficient way of obtaining answers to your own questions can lead to problems in effective diagnosis by preventing you from considering the wider picture. Questioning skills used inappropriately (process) can lead directly to poor hypothesis generation (perceptual):

Compare
Patient: *'I've been having to get up in the night to pass water lately.'*
Doctor: *'OK. How many times each night? Is there a poor stream? Is it difficult to start the flow? Do you dribble afterwards?' etc.*

with
Patient: *'I've been having to get up in the night to pass water lately.'*
Doctor: *'Yes ...'*
Patient: *'And I've been drinking a lot.'*

Doctor: *'Ah ha.'*
Patient: *'My mother's diabetic, do you think I could be?'*

EXAMPLE 2

It is fascinating to examine the link between inner thoughts and feelings and outward communication. Thoughts and feelings about a patient (perceptual) can interfere with our normal behaviour and block our communication. For instance:

- irritation with a patient's personality (perceptual) can interfere with listening and lead us to miss important cues (process)
- physical attraction to a patient (perceptual) can prevent us from asking questions about sexual matters (content) that are vital to making a correct diagnosis.

EXAMPLE 3

Unchecked erroneous assumptions (perceptual) can block effective information gathering (process) and lead us into the wrong area for discussion (content). For instance, assuming that a patient has come back for a routine check of an ongoing problem can prevent us from finding out until late in the proceedings that the patient has a more important problem or new symptom to discuss.

Too often these three types of skills have been artificially divided in medical education to the detriment of learners. In undergraduate medicine, content skills, such as the important closed questions to ask a patient with a clinical history suggestive of a heart complaint, may be taught in a history-taking course by hospital specialists. 'Communication' may be taught in a totally different course that concentrates solely on the process skills; it may be taught primarily by general practitioners and psychiatrists. This can give inappropriate messages to learners about the bona fide nature of communication as a clinical skill: 'real' doctors teach 'real' medicine and are not interested in communication skills; namby-pamby doctors teach namby-pamby medicine and cannot take a clinical history. The message goes out that 'communication is not important in the real world'.

Clearly, content, process and perceptual skills must be integrated in our teaching: all are essential clinical skills. They should be taught together, taking a wider view of the communication syllabus than has sometimes been done in the past when only process (or content) skills were considered. In Chapters 8 and 9 we discuss strategies for teaching the three types of skills together, integrating communication with other clinical skills throughout the medical curriculum and involving primary care physicians and other specialists in communication skills teaching.

An overall curriculum of doctor–patient communication skills

The three types of skills described above provide a broad frame of reference to work from. But what exactly are the specific skills of doctor–patient communication? How can we define the individual skills that we wish to include in the curriculum? How do we make them more readily accessible to facilitators and learners so they can understand the extent of the overall curriculum? And how can we present them so learners remember the individual skills and understand how they relate to each other and the consultation as a whole? Here we focus deliberately on process skills. Although content skills such as the questions that constitute the family history or functional enquiry are vitally important, they are well described in many traditional textbooks. It is the process skills that are less well described and most require definition and exploration here.

The *Calgary–Cambridge observation guide* to the consultation

The *Calgary–Cambridge observation guide* (Kurtz and Silverman 1996) was designed to answer the above questions in a concrete, concise and accessible format. The guide defines a skills-based curriculum based on four main elements which influence 'what to teach and learn' in communication programmes:

1 **structure:** how do we organize communication skills?
2 **skills:** what are the skills that we are trying to promote?
3 **validity:** what evidence is there that these skills make a difference to doctor–patient communication and its outcomes?
4 **breadth:** what is the scope of the communication curriculum?

The guide has two broad aims. Firstly, to help facilitators and learners conceptualize and structure their teaching and learning. Secondly, to assist communication programme directors, whether working in undergraduate, residency or continuing medical education, in their efforts to establish training programmes for both learners and facilitators.

In four pages, the guide:

- proposes a framework for organizing the skills of medical communication that corresponds directly to the way we structure the consultation and therefore aids teaching, learning and medical practice
- delineates and describes the individual skills that make up effective doctor–patient communication
- summarizes and makes more accessible the literature regarding doctor–patient communication skills
- forms the foundation of a comprehensive communication curriculum (Riccardi and Kurtz 1983; Kurtz 1989), providing learners, facilitators and programme directors alike with a clear idea of the curriculum's objectives
- provides a concise summary of the skills for both facilitators and learners which they can use on an everyday basis during teaching sessions as an accessible *aide-mémoire* and a way to structure observation, feedback and self-evaluation
- provides a common language for labelling and referring to specific behaviours
- provides a sound basis for the content of facilitator training programmes, creating coherence and consistency in the teaching of the large number of facilitators required in a communication programme
- provides a common foundation for communication programmes at all levels of training – undergraduate, residency and continuing medical education – by specifying a comprehensive set of core patient–doctor communication skills, equally valid and applicable in all three contexts.

Although in the past many people have clarified what to teach and numerous guides and checklists have been available, including our own previous versions (Stillman *et al.* 1976; Cassata 1978; Sanson-Fisher 1981; Riccardi and Kurtz 1983; Cohen-Cole 1991; van Thiel *et al.* 1991; Novack *et al.* 1992), the *Calgary–Cambridge observation guide* makes significant advances by:

- taking into account the current move to a more patient-centred and collaborative approach
- referencing the list of skills in line with current research and theory
- increasing the emphasis on the extremely important area of explanation and planning (Carroll and Monroe 1979; Riccardi and Kurtz 1983; Tuckett *et al.* 1985; Maguire *et al.* 1986*b*; Sanson-Fisher *et al.* 1991).

The guide has been carefully developed and refined over many years and in many different medical contexts. We are particularly indebted to Dr Rob Sanson-Fisher (Australia) for his contributions to the structure and skills of parts of the guide and to Drs Vincent Riccardi (USA) and Catherine Heaton (Canada) who were joint authors of earlier versions. This evolving guide has been used for the last 20 years as a central feature of the undergraduate communication curriculum at the University of Calgary Faculty of Medicine in Canada (Riccardi and Kurtz 1983; Kurtz 1989). More recently, the guide has been adapted for wider use, to include family medicine, internal medicine and other residents as well as practising physicians. It has also been introduced into the teaching of British general practice residents and their facilitators in the East Anglian region and has been refined through a process of experimentation in workshops with practising physicians and facilitators. The guide is equally suited to both small-group and one-to one-teaching.

The structure of the *Calgary–Cambridge observation guide*

The guide uses a simple five-point plan within which the individual skills are structured. This plan is based on the five basic tasks that physicians and patients routinely attempt to accomplish in everyday clinical practice. Physicians and patients tend to carry out these tasks roughly in sequence, with the exception of relationship building, a task which is performed continuously throughout the interview. The tasks therefore make intuitive sense and provide a logical organizational schema for both physician–patient interactions and communication skill education. This structure was first proposed by Riccardi and Kurtz in 1983 and is similar to that adopted by Cohen-Cole in 1991.

THE TASKS

1 **Initiating the session**
2 **Gathering information**
3 **Building the relationship**
4 **Explanation and planning**
5 **Closing the session**

An expanded framework of skill sets then provides further detail of the steps to be achieved within each part of the consultation:

THE EXPANDED FRAMEWORK

1 **Initiating the session:**
   - establishing initial rapport
   - identifying the reason(s) for the consultation
2 **Gathering information:**
   - exploration of problems
   - understanding the patient's perspective
   - providing structure to the consultation
3 **Building the relationship:**
   - developing rapport
   - involving the patient
4 **Explanation and planning:**
   - providing the correct amount and type of information
   - aiding accurate recall and understanding
   - achieving a shared understanding: incorporating the patient's perspective
   - planning: shared decision making
   - options in explanation and planning
     - if discussing opinion and significance of problems
     - if negotiating mutual plan of action
     - if discussing investigations and procedures
5 **Closing the session.**

The skills of the *Calgary–Cambridge observation guide*

The guide then lists the *individual* skills within this overall framework:

Initiating the session

Establishing initial rapport
1 Greets patient and obtains patient's name
2 Introduces self and clarifies role
3 Demonstrates interest and respect, attends to patient's physical comfort

Identifying the reason(s) for the consultation
4 The opening question: identifies the problems or issues that the patient wishes to address (e.g. 'What would you like to discuss today?')
5 Listening to the patient's opening statement: listens attentively, without interrupting or directing patient's response
6 Screening: checks and confirms list of problems (e.g. 'So that's headaches and tiredness. Is there anything else you'd like to discuss today?')
7 Agenda setting: negotiates agenda, taking both patient's and physician's needs into account

Gathering information

Exploration of problems
8 Patient's narrative: encourages patient to tell the story of the problem(s) from when first started to the present in own words (clarifying reason for presenting now)
9 Question style: uses open and closed questioning techniques, appropriately moving from open-ended to closed
10 Listening: listens attentively, allowing patient to complete statements without interruption and leaving space for patient to think before answering or go on after pausing
11 Facilitative response: facilitates patient's responses verbally and non-verbally (e.g. use of encouragement, silence, repetition, paraphrasing, interpretation)
12 Clarification: checks out statements which are vague or need amplification (e.g. 'Could you explain what you mean by light-headed?')
13 Internal summary: periodically summarizes to verify own understanding of what the patient has said; invites patient to correct interpretation or provide further information
14 Language: uses concise, easily understood questions and comments, avoids or adequately explains jargon

Understanding the patient's perspective
15 Ideas and concerns: determines and acknowledges patient's ideas (i.e. beliefs re cause) and concerns (i.e. worries) regarding each problem
16 Effects: determines how each problem affects the patient's life
17 Expectations: determines patient's goals, what help the patient had expected for each problem
18 Feelings and thoughts: encourages expression of the patient's feelings and thoughts
19 Cues: picks up verbal and non-verbal cues (body language, speech, facial expression, affect); checks out and acknowledges as appropriate

Providing structure to the consultation

20 Internal summary: summarizes at the end of a specific line of inquiry to confirm understanding before moving on to the next section

21 Signposting: progresses from one section to another using transitional statements; includes rationale for next section

22 Sequencing: structures interview in logical sequence

23 Timing: attends to timing and keeping interview on task

Building the relationship

Developing rapport

24 Non-verbal behaviour: demonstrates appropriate non-verbal behaviour (e.g. eye contact, posture and position, movement, facial expression, use of voice)

25 Use of notes: if reads, writes notes or uses computer, does in a manner that does not interfere with dialogue or rapport

26 Acceptance: acknowledges patient's views and feelings; accepts legitimacy; is not judgemental

27 Empathy and support: expresses concern, understanding, willingness to help; acknowledges coping efforts and appropriate self-care

28 Sensitivity: deals sensitively with embarrassing and disturbing topics and physical pain, including when associated with physical examination

Involving the patient

29 Sharing of thoughts: shares thinking with patient as appropriate to encourage patient's involvement, enhance understanding (e.g. 'What I'm thinking now is ...')

30 Provides rationale: explains rationale for questions or parts of physical examination that could appear to be non-sequiturs

31 Examination: during physical examination, explains process, asks permission

Explanation and planning

Providing the correct amount and type of information

Aims: to give comprehensive and appropriate information
         to assess each individual patient's information needs
         to neither restrict nor overload

32 Chunks and checks: gives information in assimilable chunks; checks for understanding, uses patient's response as a guide to how to proceed

33 Assesses patient's starting point: asks for patient's prior knowledge early on when giving information; discovers extent of patient's wish for information

34 Asks patients what other information would be helpful (e.g. aetiology, prognosis)

35 Gives explanation at appropriate times: avoids giving advice, information or reassurance prematurely

Aiding accurate recall and understanding

Aims: to make information easier for the patient to remember and understand

36 Organizes explanation: divides into discrete sections; develops a logical sequence

37 Uses explicit categorization or signposting (e.g. 'There are three important things that I would like to discuss. First ...'; 'Now, shall we move on to ...')
38 Uses repetition and summarizing to reinforce information
39 Language: uses concise, easily understood statements; avoids or explains jargon
40 Uses visual methods of conveying information: diagrams, models, written information and instructions
41 Checks patient's understanding of information given (or plans made), e.g. by asking patient to restate in own words; clarifies as necessary

Achieving a shared understanding: incorporating the patient's perspective
Aims: to provide explanations and plans that relate to the patient's perspective of the problem
to discover the patient's thoughts and feelings about the information given
to encourage an interaction rather than one-way transmission

42 Relates explanations to patient's illness framework: to previously elicited ideas, concerns and expectations
43 Provides opportunities and encourages patient to contribute: to ask questions, seek clarification or express doubts; responds appropriately
44 Picks up verbal and non-verbal cues, e.g. patient's need to contribute information or ask questions; information overload; distress
45 Elicits patient's beliefs, reactions and feelings re information given, terms used; acknowledges and addresses where necessary

Planning: shared decision making
Aims: to allow patients to understand the decision-making process
to involve patients in decision making to the level they wish
to increase patients' commitment to plans made

46 Shares own thoughts: ideas, thought processes and dilemmas as appropriate
47 Involves patient by making suggestions rather than directives
48 Encourages patient to contribute their thoughts: ideas, suggestions and preferences
49 Negotiates a mutually acceptable plan
50 Offers choices: encourages patient to make choices and decisions to the level that they wish
51 Checks with patient: if plans accepted; if concerns have been addressed

Closing the session

52 End summary: summarizes session briefly and clarifies plan of care
53 Contracting: contracts with patient re next steps for patient and physician
54 Safety netting: explains possible unexpected outcomes; what to do if plan is not working; when and how to seek help
55 Final checking: checks that patient agrees and is comfortable with plan and asks if any corrections, questions or other items to discuss

Options in explanation and planning

If discussing opinion and significance of problems
56 Offers opinion of what is going on and names if possible

57 Reveals rationale for opinion
58 Explains causation, seriousness, expected outcome, short- and long-term consequences
59 Elicits patient's beliefs, reactions and concerns, e.g. if opinion matches patient's thoughts, acceptability, feelings

If negotiating mutual plan of action
60 Discusses options, e.g. no action, investigation, medication or surgery; non-drug treatments [physiotherapy, walking aids, fluids, counselling]; preventative measures
61 Provides information on action or treatment offered, e.g. name; steps involved; how it works; benefits and advantages; possible side-effects
62 Obtains patient's view of need for action, perceived benefits, barriers, motivation
63 Accepts patient's views; advocates alternative viewpoint as necessary
64 Elicits patient's reactions and concerns about plans and treatments, including acceptability
65 Takes patient's lifestyle, beliefs, cultural background and abilities into consideration
66 Encourages patient to be involved in implementing plans, to take responsibility and be self-reliant
67 Asks about patient support systems; discusses other support available

If discussing investigations and procedures
68 Provides clear information on procedures, including what patient might experience and how patient will be informed of results
69 Relates procedures to treatment plan: value and purpose
70 Encourages questions about, and discussion of, potential anxieties or negative outcomes

The need for a structure

An important element of the curriculum that we have described above is the provision of a clear, overall structure within which the individual communication skills are organized. We refer to this conceptual framework repeatedly in both this and our companion book. Why do we place such importance on defining such an overt structure?

An understanding of the structure has benefits for practitioners, learners and facilitators alike.

- **For practitioners,** an awareness of the structure prevents the consultation from wandering aimlessly and important points from being missed. Communication skills are not used randomly: different skills need to be deployed purposefully and intentionally at different points in the consultation. Keeping the structure in mind helps us to remain aware of the distinct phases of the interview as we proceed. For instance, without recognizing that the gathering-information phase of the interview involves developing an understanding of the patient's individual reaction to their illness as well as the clinical aspects of their disease, the doctor may enter the explanation and planning phase of the interview prematurely and fail to address the patient's real concerns. Of course, an awareness of structure in the consultation has to be combined with flexibility: consultations do not have a fixed path that can be dictated by the doctor without reference to the patient. But without structure, it is all too easy for communication to be unsystematic and unproductive.
- **For learners at all levels,** a list of the individual communication skills alone is not sufficient. There are too many skills to remember if they are simply listed without categorization. Learners need an overall conceptual framework to help organize the skills into a memorable and useful whole. In Chapter 3 we discuss the importance of experiential methods in producing change in learners' communication skills. Experiential learning is, however, intrinsically random and opportunistic – the feedback and suggestions can be difficult to pull together. Providing a structure into which skills can be placed as they arise helps learners to order the skills that they discover opportunistically in experiential work and to see how the individual pieces fit together into the consultation as a whole.
- **Facilitators** may also lack a clear idea of how to pull together the individual skills or skill sets that they recognize as important learning areas. Without an overall framework, the numerous skills of the medical interview can appear to be a disorganized bag of tricks. Facilitators can find it difficult to link the different skills together in their teaching. A clear and overt structure can help overcome this problem. Structure has the added advantage of enabling facilitators to take an outcome-based approach in their communication skills teaching (see Chapter 5). Structure establishes an overview, enabling facilitators to ask two central questions of learners: 'Where are you in the interview?' and 'What are you and the patient trying to achieve?'. Having established a direction, the individual skills then help with the next question, 'How might you get there?'.

We use the framework to structure our communication learning and effort in much the same way that experienced clinicians use schema in clinical reasoning: to access and apply knowledge or skills systematically, to aid memory, to impose coherence and order on what would otherwise be unusable and random pieces of information.

Choosing the skills to include in the communication curriculum

We are well aware that the extensive list of skills included in the guide can initially be rather daunting to new learners and facilitators. We can almost hear readers saying 'You must be joking. Seventy skills to learn, assimilate and master: that's impossible!'. Does it really need to be that complicated? Couldn't we reduce the numbers or amalgamate a few items? Is it really necessary to try to incorporate all these skills into each consultation?

Our unapologetic answer to this is that the medical interview is indeed very complex and cannot be summed up in a few broad generalizations. We have already seen in Chapter 1 that communication is a series of learned skills and that it is both possible and essential to break the consultation down into these individual skills if we wish to identify, practise and assimilate new behaviours into our practice of medicine. All of the skills listed in the guide can be of great value to the process of the interview, all, as we will see below, have been validated by theory or research and all will repay our attention.

However, we are not suggesting that every skill needs to be employed on every occasion. By making this clear to learners from the outset, we can help defuse the anxiety associated with such a large list. For instance, although most of the skills in the gathering-information phase of the interview are appropriate to every consultation, the use of many of the items in the explanation and planning phase needs to be tailored to the individual circumstances of the interview – they will not be used in every consultation. Nonetheless, familiarity with all of the skills will undoubtedly benefit learners. At the very least, they can then be used intentionally and deliberately whenever the going gets tough!

But what is the basis for the inclusion of each of the 70 listed skills in the Calgary–Cambridge curriculum? Are we able to validate the importance of each of these skills in any way or is it purely subjective opinion? Where does the justification for these particular skills come from?

The research and theoretical bases that validate the inclusion of each individual skill

It is no longer appropriate to consider communication skills teaching as simply raising awareness of the importance of communication in the consultation. Nor is it just a matter of sharing various approaches, increasing the range of possibilities available or treating all suggestions as equally valid. Certain skills and methods have now been shown to make a substantial difference to doctor–patient communication and to ensuing health outcomes.

We are fortunate that over the last 25 years an extensive canon of theoretical and research evidence has accumulated which enables us to define the skills that enhance communication between patient and physician. Research clearly demonstrates how the use of specific skills can lead to improvements in patient satisfaction, adherence, symptom relief and physiological outcome. We can now promote these skills as worth teaching and encouraging within a communication programme. We are able confidently to answer the question 'Where's the validity?' and effectively counter the suggestion that communication skills are purely subjective.

The curriculum of skills is not and should not be static: research will continue to accumulate to challenge our preconceptions and move the goalposts of communication skills teaching. For instance, in recent years research findings have enabled the curriculum to shift in two important directions. Firstly, there has been increasing emphasis on the important but often previously neglected field of explanation and planning (information giving). Secondly, there has been a gradual move towards a more patient-centred and collaborative approach.

In this chapter, we have simply delineated a curriculum for communication skills programmes by listing and briefly defining each skill. In our companion title, *Skills for Communicating with Patients*, we describe the skills more fully and examine in depth the concepts, principles and research evidence that validate each skill.

The underlying principles of communication that have helped guide us in choosing the skills

As well as the research evidence, three immediate *goals* (Box 2.1) and five *principles* of communication (Box 2.2) also influenced the choice of skills to include in the guide. Together, they combine to provide a simple and coherent theoretical foundation for the guide and for the development of communication curricula in general.

Box 2.1 Goals of medical communication

The three immediate goals that physicians attempt to achieve whenever they talk to patients are:

1 accuracy
2 efficiency
3 supportiveness.

Effective communication provides the means of accomplishing these goals (Riccardi and Kurtz 1983).

Box 2.2 Principles that characterize effective communication

The following five principles, applicable to any setting, help us to understand what constitutes effective communication (Kurtz 1989).

Effective communication:

1 *ensures an interaction rather than a direct transmission process.* If communication is viewed as a direct transmission process, the senders of messages can assume that their responsibilities as communicators are fulfilled once they have formulated and sent a message. However, if communication is viewed as an interactive process, the interaction is complete only if the sender receives feedback about how the message is interpreted, whether it is understood and what impact it has on the receiver. Just imparting information or just listening is not enough: giving and receiving feedback about the impact of the message becomes crucial. The emphasis moves to the interdependence of sender and receiver, and the contributions and initiatives of each become more equal in importance (Dance and Larson 1972). The aim of communication becomes the establishment of mutually understood common ground (Baker 1955).

2 *reduces unnecessary uncertainty.* It is important to consider all possible causes of uncertainty in the medical interview. Unresolved uncertainties in any area can lead to lack of concentration or anxiety which in turn can block effective communication. For example, patients may be uncertain about what to expect during a given interview, about the significance of a line of questioning, about the role of a particular member of the health care team or about the attitudes, intentions or trustworthiness of the interviewer. Reducing uncertainty about diagnosis or expected outcomes of care is obviously important although living with some uncertainty is often a necessity in medical situations. However, even then, openly discussing areas where knowledge is lacking or no one is certain of the best choice can help reduce uncertainty by establishing mutually understood common ground.

3 *requires planning and thinking in terms of outcomes.* The best way to determine effectiveness is to think in terms of outcomes and consequences. If I am angry and the outcome I seek is to vent emotion, I proceed in one direction. However, if the outcome I want is to resolve any problem or misunderstanding that may have caused my anger, I must proceed in a different way to be effective.

4 *demonstrates dynamism.* What is appropriate for one situation is inappropriate for another – different individuals' needs and contexts change continually. What the patient understood so clearly yesterday seems beyond comprehension today. Just as one area of understanding seems to be nearing completion, another avenue opens up. Dynamism underscores the need not only for *flexibility* but also for *responsiveness* and *involvement*.

5 *follows the helical model.* The helical model of communication (Dance 1967) has two implications. Firstly, what I say influences what you say in spiral fashion so that our communication gradually evolves as we interact. Secondly, reiteration and repetition, coming back around the spiral of communication at a slightly different level each time, are essential for effective communication.

Summary

In this chapter we have defined the broad categories of skills that constitute medical communication. We have described the individual skills to be included in communication curricula and have discussed the theoretical and research bases that validate the choice of these particular skills. We have presented the curriculum of skills in the form of the *Calgary–Cambridge observation guide* which not only lists the skills but also provides a structure or conceptual framework that enables facilitators and learners to make sense of the individual skills and how they relate to the consultation as a whole.

The skills collated in the guide provide the foundations for effective doctor–patient communication in many different medical contexts. The guide is comprehensive but not all-encompassing: there are circumstances in which additional issue-specific skills are also required such as in breaking bad news, bereavement, revealing hidden depression, gender and cultural issues, prevention and motivation (Gask *et al.* 1988; Maguire and Faulkner 1988*a*; Sanson-Fisher *et al.* 1991; Chugh *et al.* 1993). These issues clearly deserve special attention in our teaching and we explore them further in both this and our companion volume. However, we stress that the skills delineated in the guide are the *core* communication skills required in all these circumstances, providing a secure platform on which specific communication issues and challenges can be superimposed.

The guide does not just summarize the 'what' of the communication curriculum, it is an important part of the 'how' of communication skills teaching too. Throughout this book we repeatedly return to the guide which is the centrepiece of our whole approach to communication skills teaching. We explore how:

- both facilitators and learners can use the guide as a concise, usefully organized and readily accessible *aide-mémoire* which they can refer to easily during observation, feedback, self-evaluation and discussion sessions. The guide helps make learning more systematic
- the guide helps to organize and structure learning over time by enabling facilitators and learners to summarize and keep track of opportunistic learning and to piece together randomly identified skills as they arise throughout the helical curriculum. It allows facilitators and learners to place skills and information covered in any particular consultation or teaching session in context and to make a record of areas explored during a given teaching session or over the course as a whole. The guide counters the random nature of skills work in problem-based, experiential learning by providing a framework within which to place these individual skills and build up a coherent overall schema
- the guide can be used in both formative and summative assessment. Using the guide as the basis for self, peer and formal or certifying evaluation encourages an open understanding between course directors and students without the possibility of hidden agendas (Heaton and Kurtz 1992*ab*)
- with only slight adjustment to format, the guide can be used across all levels of medical education, from undergraduate to residency and continuing medical education, and can therefore provide a common foundation for communication programmes at all these levels.

3

The 'how': principles of how to teach and learn communication skills

Introduction

We have established that:

- there is a need to teach and learn communication in medicine
- communication can be taught
- communication training makes a difference
- we can define and structure a curriculum of communication skills.

But *how* do you actually teach and learn communication skills? Can we say which teaching methods work in practice? Is there evidence that any particular methods are more helpful than others or is it all subjective opinion?

There is a clear parallel here between the consultation and teaching and learning communication skills. We have already demonstrated that knowing 'what' to say or do in the medical interview is not enough; 'how' you communicate is equally important. Similarly, knowing 'what' to teach and learn in communication programmes is an essential first step but success is critically dependent on 'how' we do things.

The remainder of this book explores the 'how' of communication skills teaching and learning in considerable depth. In this chapter we provide an overview that enables readers to see the 'big picture' and to gain a broad understanding of the principles underpinning this complex subject before delving into any one area more deeply. We explore four questions which help to frame everything that follows:

1 Why take a skills-based approach to communication teaching and learning?
  - the importance of both skills and attitudinal approaches to communication teaching
  - the rationale for taking a predominantly skills-based approach

2 Why is it necessary to learn communication skills experientially?
- the evidence that experiential learning is necessary to achieve change
- the essential ingredients of experiential communication skills learning

3 Why take a problem-based approach and adhere to adult learning principles?
- the relevance of adult learning principles to communication skills training
- using a problem-based approach in experiential communication skills learning
- the balance between self-directed and facilitator-directed learning

4 Why complement experiential learning with didactic methods and cognitive material?
- why include didactic teaching in the communication skills programme?

Why take a skills-based approach to communication teaching and learning?

This book takes a predominantly skills-based approach to communication. The teaching and learning methods that we advocate are very much geared towards specific skills acquisition. Is this position justified?

The importance of both skills and attitudinal approaches to communication teaching

There has been much debate about how to approach the teaching of communication between doctors and patients. The argument revolves around how exactly to bridge the gulf between doctors' actual behaviour in the consultation and the behaviours that we know can make a positive difference to outcomes for both patient and doctor. Where does the block lie and what is the best way to overcome it? At its most polarized there appear to be two very different and, at first sight, mutually exclusive viewpoints which dominate the discussion, with proponents dividing into separate 'attitudes' and 'skills' camps. We know that physicians' attitudes and skills tend to go together – for example, Levinson and Roter (1995) have shown that physicians with positive attitudes to psychosocial aspects of patient care use more patient-centred skills and have more collaborative relationships with their patients. But how do we influence learners to move in this direction – through training in skills or attitudes? The question is not purely academic. The teaching methods of attitudinal and skills work are very different: how we teach communication is critically dependent upon which approach we take.

THE SKILLS APPROACH

The rationale behind the skills approach to communication teaching may be summarized as follows:

- communication is a skill
- it is a series of learned skills and not simply a matter of personality
- individual skills can be delineated and learned
- knowledge of appropriate skills does not translate directly to performance

- practice with observation and feedback is required to achieve acquisition of new skills and change in learners' behaviour
- communication training requires 'formal' instruction that is intentional, systematic, specific and experiential.

Skills teaching seeks to improve the performance of learners' communication skills. It attempts to help learners not only to gain an understanding of *what* the appropriate communication skills are in different parts of the interview but also to learn *how* to incorporate these behaviours into their everyday practice. It breaks down the performance as a whole into its constituent parts, into specific skills and behaviours that can be separately practised and rehearsed (Pacoe *et al.* 1976). The message here is that although understanding what it takes to communicate effectively is important, to actually improve communication it is essential to be able to use communication skills in practice. The difference is between understanding and doing. Learners need the opportunity to practise the appropriate skills so that they become part of their repertoire and can be used appropriately and intentionally whenever the situation dictates. New skills need to be worked on in safety until learners feel comfortable using them in the consultation. The skills approach helps learners to acquire the numerous skills that research and experience have shown to aid doctor–patient communication and to incorporate them into their own style.

THE ATTITUDE APPROACH

In contrast, the 'attitude' approach says that the block to communication does not lie primarily with poor skills but at a deeper level of attitudes and emotions. Proponents of this argument suggest that doctors may well have appropriate skills and be using them already in circumstances outside medicine. However, they are not transferring the use of these skills to the consulting room because of important blocks in their relationship with patients that need to be overcome before any progress can be made. Many of these attitudinal problems relate to the institution of medicine itself, to doctors' previous educational experiences and to the behaviour of the role models that they observe within the system. Perhaps the fundamental question here relates to the doctors' beliefs about the roles of patients and doctors in the therapeutic process. Consider the doctor who has a disease-orientated, doctor-centred attitude to patients in which patients' views are not appreciated as being important and emotional issues are avoided. According to this approach, only when these restrictive attitudinal blocks have been confronted and changed will the doctor be able to relate appropriately and communicate effectively with his patients. Learning therefore concentrates on an exploration of the doctor's thoughts, feelings and emotions towards patients, exploring where these are coming from and whether they are productive or counter-productive to the doctor–patient interaction.

WHY BOTH SKILLS AND ATTITUDES?

Of course, the truth lies somewhere between the two extreme positions of this debate. Skills and attitudes are both important, both must be addressed, both demand careful attention. In fact, they share much more common ground than is apparent at first sight. The two approaches are linked together by the concept of outcome. One of the principles of communication that we discussed in Chapter 2 is that effective communication is outcome based (Kurtz 1989). The most effective way to behave in a given situation is dependent on what you want to achieve. So, as described in detail in Chapter 5, in skills-based teaching we encourage learners first to identify what they are aiming for. Only then can they choose the skills that will help them get to where they want to go. Attitudinal work is part of this process of examining objectives – it simply takes the idea one step further back. It encourages learners to explore the outcomes they are aiming for by examining the very roots of their relationships with patients and what it is that they and the patients are trying to achieve during the consultation.

So why take a predominantly skills-based approach?

If skills and attitudes both merit our attention in communication skills programmes, why does this book advocate a predominantly skills-based approach to communication teaching and learning?

1 *Skills acquisition is the one essential component of communication teaching and learning.* Although increased understanding and insight are readily achieved through attitudinal work, learners can only acquire the skills to translate this understanding into practice through a skills-based approach. It may, for instance, become apparent through attitudinal work that increased empathy towards the patient might enable a learner to achieve more in the consultation. But the learner may have little idea how to put this concept into practice. Without carrying attitudinal work one essential step further into skills acquisition, learners often cannot convert their new-found intentions into appropriate behaviour.

The skills approach is the final common pathway for improving communication in practice and although attitude work is important in raising awareness and increasing the desire to change skills, it may well be impotent in effecting useful change in learners' behaviour without the addition of skills training.

2 *Skills acquisition is important even where there are no attitudinal blocks.* Even where there are no problems at all at an attitudinal level, there is still a need to explore and assimilate communication skills that will help learners be more effective in the consultation. We can all think of people with all the 'right' attitudes and intentions but with hopeless interpersonal skills. All of us can improve and refine our skills whatever our starting point.

Even if we do use appropriate skills in different areas of our lives outside the medical arena, we may never have analysed what we do and so cannot intentionally transfer these skills into a medical context. The skills of medical communication are often not apparent at first sight nor are they exactly the same as the skills we use in other relationships. We may, for instance, appreciate the value of fully understanding the patient's story from their own perspective but it may not be immediately obvious that summarizing is one of the key skills in information gathering and relationship building that enables us to achieve this aim. Similarly, how intuitive is it that the facilitative response of repetition is actually counter-productive in the early stages of the interview but of great benefit later on?

3 *The skills approach is less threatening to the defensive learner.* For the less motivated learner, 'the reluctant traveller', tackling skills rather than attitudes can be less threatening and therefore more likely to achieve change. Imagine the doctor who has been practising medicine for

20 years and is challenged in discussion to consider whether his paternalistic attitude to patients throughout that time has been appropriate. It almost invites the defensive reply 'My attitude's fine, thank you very much'. Taking a more skills-based approach to, say, patient non-compliance and discussing and practising the skills of eliciting patients' expectations in that context can be far less threatening. There is a big difference between suggesting someone change their attitude and offering them a skill that will help them achieve an outcome they already have in mind.

4 *Skills acquisition can lead to changes in attitude.* In our experience, you do not have to alter attitudes first before new skills can be assimilated. On the contrary, the acquisition of skills can open the path to changes in attitude. For instance, a doctor may learn and assimilate the skill of active listening at the beginning of the consultation to help improve his hypothesis generation. As a consequence of using this skill, more statements and clues to the patient's ideas, concerns and expectations will appear. The doctor's consultations will be altered as he begins to hear and address the patient's concerns. This change may lead him to understand the importance of a less disease-centred approach and to appreciate the difference that understanding patients' needs can make to the effectiveness of his work. The application of a skill may therefore lead to a change in attitudes and beliefs.

Perhaps an analogy would be useful.* Imagine the skills of medical communication to be a set of tools in a mechanic's tool-box. Each tool is purpose made to accomplish a particular task elegantly and efficiently. No doubt, you can remove a nut with a hammer and chisel but how much more satisfying, time saving and safe to do it with a well-polished socket wrench. Practice is required to learn which tasks are best achieved with which tool and how to use each one most effectively.

The mechanic does not use all the tools all the time but in a difficult situation he knows where to find just the right tool for the job. It helps for the tool-box to have compartments (analogous to the structure of the consultation). The sections of the tool-box help the mechanic to organize his tools so he knows where they are and which tools work well together.

Of course, just having the tools is not enough. A mechanic without appropriate attitudes will not suddenly become an expert just because he has been given a tool kit for his birthday. He has to have a feel for cars and enjoy working on them. He needs knowledge of car maintenance and servicing. He has to practise with the tools until he masters their use and look after them if they get dull or rusty. Without this feel for car maintenance and appreciation of tools, he is unlikely to use the tools to their best advantage. Attitudes and skills go hand in hand. Being given the right tools may well be the spur to develop further an appreciation for car maintenance. But becoming aware of the value of car maintenance can be a recipe for frustration unless we provide the opportunity for obtaining the appropriate tools as well.

Skills versus issues

Communication programmes can also take an issues-based approach in which coursework is organized around issues such as ethics, culture, age, death and dying and addiction. Again we

* We are grateful to Sue Weaver for suggesting this analogy.

advocate taking a predominantly skills-based approach rather than an issues-based approach. The core skills of the *Calgary–Cambridge observation guide* presented in Chapter 2 are of fundamental importance. They provide the foundations for effective doctor–patient communication in many different medical contexts and supply a secure platform on which specific communication issues and challenges can be superimposed. Once core skills are mastered, specific communication issues are much more readily tackled.

Our approach is therefore to expend more effort on core skills than issues. Although issues are highly important and must be included in the communication programme, we prefer not to base our teaching around an exploration of each separate issue as if it were a completely new problem unrelated to core skills. Instead we find it more effective to use such issues to illustrate relevant components of a skills-based curriculum, to demonstrate how core skills can be employed in specific circumstances and what issue-specific skills need to be superimposed upon them.

The well-rounded communication curriculum deals with skills, attitudes and specific communication issues. In Chapter 8 we explore how to combine the teaching of these three areas and, in particular, how to include the teaching of attitudes and issues within a predominantly skills-based curriculum.

Which teaching and learning methods work in practice?

Having established the rationale for taking a predominantly skills-based approach, we now examine the research evidence showing that certain methods are necessary for communication training to bear fruit. Together, three complementary approaches maximize learning in communication skills training:

1 experiential learning methods
2 problem-based learning methods
3 didactic methods.

Why use experiential learning methods?

In Chapter 1 we presented the research evidence showing that communication skills in medicine can be taught. But what teaching methods did these various studies use to bring about such impressive changes in learners' communication skills? Table 3.1 summarizes the approaches taken in each paper.

The communication skills programmes described in these papers relied heavily on experiential rather than didactic methods of learning. In particular, almost all used video or audio recordings of interviews with real or simulated patients followed by observation and feedback. But are these experiential methods necessary for learning communication? Do we know that traditional apprenticeship or didactic teaching methods by themselves will not bring about the same changes in behaviours and skills? Why when experiential methods are

Table 3.1 Teaching methods used to bring about changes in learners' communication skills

	Handouts	Lectures	Training workshop	Video/ audio rec	Real patients	Simulated patients	Role play	Feedback
Rutter and Maguire (1976)	✓			✓	✓			✓
Irwin and Bamber (1984)				✓	✓			✓
Evans et al. (1989, 1991)		✓		✓	✓	✓	✓	✓
Stillman et al. (1976, 1977)				✓		✓		✓
Sanson-Fisher and Poole (1978)			✓					
Putnam et al. (1988)	✓		✓	✓	✓			✓
Joos et al. (1996)	✓	✓	✓	✓		✓		✓
Goldberg et al. (1980)				✓	✓			✓
Gask et al. (1987, 1988)	✓			✓	✓			✓
Levinson and Roter (1993)	✓	✓		✓	✓	✓	✓	✓
Inui et al. (1976)			✓					
Roter et al. (1995)	✓	✓	✓	✓	✓		✓	✓

potentially more challenging, threatening and less safe for the learner do we insist on their use? Isn't knowledge of the skills enough without having to practise them as well?

The evidence that specific experiential learning methods are necessary

The evidence that we now present serves to underline the significant difference between knowing about the skills and behaviours that comprise effective communication and being able to put these skills into practice. Knowledge does not translate directly to performance: a further step of specific experiential work is required to acquire new skills and change learners' behaviour.

> *I hear and I forget*
> *I see and I remember*
> *I do and I understand*
>   Old Chinese proverb

Perhaps the most significant studies here are those of Maguire *et al*. Their initial work showed that medical students who underwent an interview training programme in history-taking skills during their psychiatry clerkship reported almost three times as much relevant and accurate information after a test interview as those who received only the traditional apprenticeship method of learning history-taking skills (Rutter and Maguire 1976).

Maguire later took this research further to try to isolate which specific aspects of this interview training programme were responsible for the considerable gain in skills observed (Maguire *et al*. 1978). This work has helped guide the development of communication skills programmes ever since. He randomized medical students into four training conditions:

- group 1: traditional apprenticeship alone

- groups 2, 3, 4: the above plus discussion with a tutor of two handouts detailing areas of information to be obtained and techniques to follow
- group 2: the above plus personal feedback with a tutor on an interview that the tutor had observed on videotape and rated on a rating scale. The student did not see the recording himself
- group 3: as group 2 but here the tutor and student watched the videotape together and used this as the vehicle for giving feedback
- group 4: as group 3 but with the use of audio rather than videotape.

Each student in groups 2, 3 and 4 was given feedback on three occasions before post-training interviews were recorded to assess improvement in skills. The results showed that despite teaching received in their clinical rotations, students in group 1 showed no improvement in the amount of information elicited or in skills used. Students in all three groups who received feedback from the tutor showed significant gains in the amount of information obtained but only students in groups 3 and 4 who had received the benefit of audio or videotape feedback showed significant gain in their communication skills. All results favoured the video over the audio group although not at statistically significant levels.

Roe (1980), working with Maguire's team, has since demonstrated that these results in one-to-one teaching are also obtained in small groups. This study also showed that it was important for a tutor who understood the model being taught to be present. Individuals or groups who watched videotapes of their own performance without the presence of a tutor and who provided their own feedback made significantly less progress than when a tutor was present.

Maguire's conclusions were that traditional medical training in communication has two major deficiencies. Firstly, there is a lack of a suitable model which makes explicit which areas medical students should cover and what skills they should use. Secondly, there is little opportunity for students to receive any systematic feedback about their ability to communicate with patients. The teaching method that he therefore suggests includes the following key steps:

- the provision of detailed, written guidelines of the areas to cover and the skills to use
- the opportunity to practise interviewing under controlled conditions
- observation by both self and facilitator
- the provision of feedback by an experienced facilitator with the aid of audio or videotape.

Evans et al. (1989) also demonstrated significant improvements in interview skills and techniques following a history-taking skills course compared to traditional medical school teaching. Again, they were able to isolate whether it was the didactic or experiential part of their teaching that actually led to change. Their course had two components:

1 a series of five one-hour lectures covering the background to communication training and the verbal, non-verbal and listening skills that were helpful in the medical interview. Students were given comprehensive handouts, including relevant theory and research
2 three two-hour workshops, after the lectures, using experiential methods such as role play, discussion, videotaping with real and simulated patients and feedback.

The results showed that although there was some improvement after the lecture series, most significant gains in history-taking skills were obtained following the small-group skills workshops.

What do these research studies tell us about how to teach and learn communication skills? They clearly demonstrate the deficiencies of the traditional apprenticeship model but they also show us that didactic methods by themselves are not sufficient to achieve change in learners' behaviour. Observation, feedback and video or audio recording of performance are required to effect improvement in learners' skills (Carroll and Monroe 1979; Simpson *et al.* 1991).

MODELLING

Does the traditional apprenticeship model have anything to offer learners in developing their communication skills? At this point we need to consider the importance of modelling. All facilitators and practising doctors observed by learners or colleagues are modelling skills, behaviours and attitudes. Modelling can have a profound effect on attitude (Siegler *et al.* 1987; Bandura 1988; Ficklin 1988). However, although it may change attitudes, by itself modelling is not sufficient to ensure that learners can identify the skills that they see, much less develop and use them appropriately in practice (Kurtz 1990). Often, learners comment on a mentor being particularly skilled at communicating with patients but when asked what makes the mentor so good, they cannot identify exactly what he does, commenting only that he is 'gifted' with patients.

That is not to say that modelling has no influence on skills. Its value in skills learning lies in its power vicariously to reinforce – or block – the development, maintenance and application of skills. It takes a determined and aware individual to keep using communication skills that doctors in the real world beyond the classroom do not seem to value or use. Developing the ability to model communication skills at a professional level is an important responsibility for facilitators in the communication programme but also for other doctors who serve as role models for learners elsewhere.

The essential ingredients of experiential communication skills learning

These are the essential ingredients of experiential communication skills learning:

- systematic delineation and definition of essential skills
- observation
- well-intentioned, detailed and descriptive feedback
- video or audio recording and review
- practice and rehearsal of skills
- active small-group or one-to-one learning.

SYSTEMATIC DELINEATION AND DEFINITION OF ESSENTIAL SKILLS

The discussion of the *Calgary–Cambridge observation guide* in Chapter 2 deals with this requirement in detail. Without inclusion of this element, experiential learning is unlikely to be successful.

OBSERVATION

Almost all the studies quoted above employed direct observation of learners interviewing either real or simulated patients. It should not be surprising that observation has been shown to be of central importance in communication skills teaching: observation is vital in learning any skill, inside or outside medicine. Ask any group of learners about their experience of observation in learning and they immediately come up with examples from their sporting experience, from learning musical instruments, from becoming skilled in practical procedures such as painting or driving. Of course, you can learn from trial and error, by practice alone, but how much more efficient to be observed and receive feedback on your work. And how difficult to improve beyond a certain point without observation and feedback. Habits become ingrained and we become stuck in ruts of our own making, in methods that feel comfortable but that might not necessarily be the best.

Yet often doctors can remember few times in the whole of their medical training when they were directly observed interacting with patients and even fewer times when the feedback that they received was constructive and of value. This paucity of observation is a common finding in medical schools both in the UK and in North America at undergraduate and residency levels (Jason and Westberg 1982; Stillman *et al*. 1986, 1987). Observation and feedback would appear to be the missing ingredients of medical education.

When doctors have been observed in their training, it has been while attempting highly practical procedures such as lumbar punctures or chest drain insertion. We would not, for instance, dream of suggesting that aspiring surgeons learn to perform a cholecystectomy without observation. Surgeons have always learned their skills by being rigorously observed and given constant feedback on their progress. How would we feel if the surgeon about to remove our own gall-bladder had learned the procedure by reading about it, watching others do it and then being told to go off and do one and come back and report how she did? Yet this is how we traditionally teach interview skills to medical students (Davidoff 1993).

This method bears a striking resemblance to Chinese whispers. Without direct observation, the story told often bears little resemblance to the truth: the teacher only gets a filtered version of what actually happened. Self-reporting is often not detailed enough to allow the teacher to understand the problem. It is very difficult for learners to remember what happened in the heat of the moment, to be specific rather than vague. It is, of course, impossible by definition to comment on one's own blind spots. The feedback offered in response is then of little value as it may well not address the difficulties that actually occurred. How can the tennis coach give you suggestions for improvement if all he has to go on is your description of the balls thudding into the net? He needs to see your forehand action and analyse the problem before providing solutions. Feedback without observation is like treatment without diagnosis.

Observation is therefore vital for both learners and teachers. And it is just as important for experts as for beginners. How do professional athletes keep at the top of their game, how do they hone and improve their skills? The same way beginners do – by observation, analysis and feedback from their peers and coaches.

WELL-INTENTIONED, DETAILED AND DESCRIPTIVE FEEDBACK

Not only are learners rarely observed during their medical education but their experiences of feedback following observation are often highly negative. The most common memory of feedback is the ward round, frequently described as a disconcerting, even humiliating, learning situation: learners report an atmosphere of competitive rather than collaborative learning. Teachers may appear unsupportive and the feedback learners receive negative, judgemental and without useful suggestions for change. Unfortunately, learners' other main experience of observation is often of certifying examinations where the only feedback received is in the form of global ratings such as pass or fail.

Learners may rarely have experienced a learning situation involving observation where they have felt supported by a well-motivated teacher able to give non-judgemental yet constructive criticism (Ende *et al.* 1983; McKegney 1989; Westberg and Jason 1993). In the past, they may not have felt able to deliberately and willingly expose their difficulties without fear of being marked down and they may have little experience of genuine formative assessment. We therefore often have an uphill struggle to win learners over to the value of observation and feedback when all their previous experiences tell them that they will not enjoy it. Observation and feedback need careful handling if their full potential for learning is to be realized.

For learners to benefit from observation, feedback needs to be specific, detailed, non-judgemental and well intentioned. The tennis coach never just observes, he provides a supportive environment and gives positive encouragement that highlights the learner's accomplishments. At the same time he provides useful, practical and well-intentioned feedback on areas that would benefit from change. Feedback is constructive: it is specific and detailed enough for learners to see how to alter their behaviour and develop their skills. Feedback is well intentioned and is provided for the benefit of the learner: the coach is there to help and encourage learners, not to demonstrate either how unskilled the learner is or how skilled the teacher.

Because descriptive feedback is central to communication skills teaching, we discuss it in depth in Chapter 5.

VIDEO AND AUDIO RECORDING AND REVIEW

It is not surprising that research highlights the importance of video and audio recordings in communication skills teaching. Learning any skill is greatly helped by self-observation, by being able to see for ourselves exactly what we are doing and where improvements might be made. In sports coaching, it is now commonplace to use video recording to enable learners as well as coaches to gain insight and learn from observation.

The use of video or audio recording to guide feedback offers many advantages over the provision of feedback from observation of the live interaction alone (Hargie and Morrow 1986; Premi 1991; Heaton and Kurtz 1992*b*; Beckman and Frankel 1994; Westberg and Jason 1994):

- learners who can observe or listen to themselves understand their own strengths and weaknesses much more readily than if they rely on reflection alone: our own perceptions of our behaviour are not always accurate
- recordings encourage a learner-centred approach with the learner being more centrally and actively involved in the analysis of the interview. Seeing themselves enables learners to make more accurate, detailed and objective self-assessments. Sharing this self-assessment is an important aspect of consultation analysis
- recordings help prevent misconceptions and disagreements over what actually occurred from getting in the way of learning. Accuracy and reliability of feedback is greatly increased

- recordings allow feedback to be much more specific as there is always an exact referent for any particular item of discussion. The tape allows learners to revisit particular points in the interview and to gain a deeper understanding of the use of exact phrasing or behaviour
- recordings help feedback to focus on description rather than evaluation, an essential aspect of constructive feedback as we shall see in Chapter 5
- recordings allow areas to be reviewed on several occasions and enable the learner to revisit feedback and learning at a later date.

Video recording has advantages over audio recording which offset the disparity in ease of use. Video makes it possible to focus feedback and self-assessment on a much broader range of non-verbal as well as verbal behaviours which could otherwise be lost to learning. Also, it is easier to concentrate for longer periods on video than on audio recordings.

PRACTICE AND REHEARSAL OF SKILLS

Practice and rehearsal are often neglected aspects of communication skills teaching and learning. Returning to our tennis analogy, good coaches do not simply make recommendations and suggest that you go away and try them out during your next competitive match. They ask you to try out new moves away from the hurly-burly of a real match and practise them repeatedly in a safe situation until you feel comfortable. They observe you as you practise new skills and give further feedback which allows you to refine your technique as you proceed.

Rehearsal in safe supportive settings is equally necessary in learning communication skills. What does rehearsal offer learners?

1 *Practising skills in safety.* It is asking too much of learners (and their patients!) to expect them to experiment with new skills for the first time in real consultations. The great selling point of experiential learning is that it can provide opportunities to practise skills in safety, where there are no adverse consequences of 'botching' an attempt at a new skill. Safe for the learner in that the setting is supportive, attempts at using skills are not subject to put-downs and risk taking and experimentation are valued. Safe for the patient who is not at risk of damage as the learner's experimentation has been done first with simulated patients or peers. What a relief to be able to say 'Well that didn't seem to work at all – can I try it again?' or 'That went well but I'd like to see what happens if I try a different approach'. The key to rehearsal is to provide safe learning opportunities which are as near as possible to real-life situations while still allowing multiple opportunities for trial and error plus feedback. We look at how to provide such safe and supportive settings for practice in more detail in Chapters 4, 5 and 6.

2 *Enabling ongoing feedback and rehearsal.* Rehearsal leads on to further observation, self and peer assessment and feedback. Feedback then leads to yet further rehearsal which enables the learner gradually to refine and master skills. It is in fact this helical, repetitive observation and feedback which so often pushes the learning process forward. Opportunities for repetitive practice and feedback need to be provided in learning situations. It is not enough simply to provide feedback without the chance to try out the suggestions that are made.

3 *Developing an individual approach.* Each learner needs to develop their own method of accomplishing a skill so that it can become incorporated into their own personality and style.

One criticism of skills-based communication skills teaching is that it is a cookbook approach that says prescriptively 'Here are the skills to be learned; this is how you should do it'. How do we reconcile the need for flexibility, individuality and personal style with the skills-based approach that we advocate in which the skills of the curriculum are so clearly defined and delineated within a 70-item guide?

The answer lies in how learners and facilitators approach these skills. Each skill listed in the guide is only a clue that this is an area where specific behaviours and phrases need to be worked on and developed experientially. The list by itself is not enough; each learner has to discover his own way to put each skill into practice. While the guides identify explicitly the skills which have emerged from research and practice as being of value in doctor–patient communication, they do not attempt to specify exact phrasing or behaviour to accomplish these skills. All they do is label the skills and sometimes offer examples. The challenge during the teaching session is to generate alternatives and to give participants the opportunity to try out and refine various phrases and behaviours without reducing flexibility or negating the influence of individual personalities. In fact, communication training should increase rather than reduce flexibility by providing an expanded repertoire of skills that physicians can adeptly and intentionally choose to use as they require.

Going beyond specific skills into individuality is the real challenge of experiential learning. We cannot be prescriptive about the best way to proceed in any circumstance. Many variables influence the choices that are best in a given situation, including the development of your own personal style. But we must also recognize that we can put forward certain reliable patterns and principles of communication, certain skills that are likely to be more effective than others, that research has proven to be of value and that will help you to be more effective and confident in the consultation.

It is practice and rehearsal that allow us to reconcile the two concepts of skills and individuality. The list of skills is only a start. To learn how to use each skill adeptly requires ongoing practice, feedback and adaptation. Through this helical, iterative process, learners stamp their own individuality on the communication process.

ACTIVE SMALL-GROUP OR ONE-TO-ONE LEARNING

Experiential learning through observation, recording, feedback and rehearsal are clearly not suited to the familiar and comfortable large group and independent study contexts used so extensively in medical education for more traditional cognitive learning. Communication skills training requires one-to-one or small-group learning in which the numbers are small enough to allow each learner frequent opportunity for practice, participation and individualized coaching.

This approach requires learners to take a more active role, to learn by doing rather than by listening or reading. Piaget's concept that you really only learn what you create or recreate for yourself is particularly relevant to communication skills programmes. Active involvement in experiential work involves a different set of learning skills than that of traditional cognitive study. This is not the world of listening to expert lectures, making notes, participating in large group discussions, studying written material and writing essays and examinations. Experiential study shifts the primary focus away from the lecture and the book to one's own behaviour. Experiential learning is more learner and less teacher centred. It is more active and less passive for learners with more time spent practising, observing and giving and receiving feedback.

Roles and responsibilities for both facilitator and learner are changed and both may need help in adapting to these new circumstances. Experiential learning can feel uncomfortable to learners and facilitators unaccustomed to this approach. Compared to didactic teaching, it can appear potentially unsafe, unstructured and random. Yet skill development does not result from listening to lectures. One of the challenges for facilitators and learners in communication skills programmes is making the transition from large-group, lecture-based teaching to small-group and one-to-one experiential learning.

Why use a problem-based approach to communication skills teaching?

So we know that learning communication skills requires specific experiential methods. But where do we start? What do we observe and why? The answer lies in a problem-based approach in which the learners' own perceived difficulties with doctor–patient communication provide the focus for observation and learning.

Why begin with learners' perceived needs? Why not simply tell them the skills they need to learn and then observe their efforts in experiential settings? Why approach communication skills from the perspective of the problems that learners are concerned with rather than from our much clearer understanding of what they and their patients actually require? After all, we have already emphasized the importance of defining the skills and producing a curriculum so why not just address learners' needs rather than their wants? The principles of adult learning (Knowles 1984) which underlie experiential learning in general and the problem-based approach in particular help to resolve this dilemma.

Adult learning

In recent years, problem-based approaches have gained increasing popularity in medical education at all levels. Knowles' principles of adult learning have been a major influence in promoting this shift. Knowles examined what motivates adults to learn and how to capitalize on this in teaching. He suggested that adult learners are motivated to learn when they perceive learning to be relevant to their current situation and when it enables them to acquire skills and knowledge which they can use in immediate and practical ways. The more relevant the learning is to the real world of their immediate experience, the more quickly and effectively adults learn. Learners are therefore motivated by a problem-based (rather than a subject-based) approach where the practical difficulties that they themselves are experiencing act as the stimulus for learning.

Building upon learners' past experiences also motivates adults to learn. Adult learners have considerable experience of the world and a great deal to offer. If their contributions are valued, accepted and used, learning will flourish; if their experience is ignored, new approaches will often be rejected out of hand.

The principles of adult learning contrast with traditional teacher-centred or didactic learning which is concerned with the direct transmission of content by the teacher to a passive learner. In problem-based learning, facilitators encourage learners to be actively involved. Not only do learners acquire knowledge, they also develop the understanding and skills to apply that knowledge in practice.

The following list characterizes what motivates adults to learn. Increasingly, medical and other educators espouse this set of ideas (for example, Barrows and Tamblyn 1981; Westberg and Jason 1993). Adults are motivated by learning which is:

- relevant to learners' present situations
- practical rather than just theoretical
- problem rather than subject centred
- built on learners' previous experience
- directed towards learners' perceived needs
- planned in terms of negotiated and emergent objectives
- participatory, actively involving learners
- geared to learners' own pace
- primarily self-directed
- designed so that learners can take responsibility for their own learning
- designed to promote more equal relationship with teachers
- evaluated through self and peer assessment.

This list is particularly relevant to communication skills teaching. Taking a problem-based approach eases the defensiveness which can accompany experiential learning. We have to remember that whether at undergraduate, residency or CME level, considerable discomfort may well ensue from entering a programme that requires you to examine and possibly change something that seems so closely bound to your personality and self-concept as communication behaviour. Experiential methods are potentially more challenging, threatening and less safe for the learner than more traditional forms of learning. It can feel uncomfortable to perform interviews while others assess your skills and, at the same time, a camera records your performance. Following the principles of adult learning can help reduce learners' defensiveness and enable them to benefit from communication training. Identifying learners' needs and discovering practical solutions to their own problems, proceeding at their pace and making the learning experience relevant to their own situation all enable learners to become less defensive and more open to learning and change.

Using a problem-based approach in practice

So to maximize learning, we not only have to use specific experiential methods, in which skills can be actively tried out and practised in a supportive environment, but also encourage a problem-based approach. Starting from where learners are, we attempt to address their needs, make learning and teaching relevant to their current situation and build on their existing knowledge, skills and experience. To prevent defensiveness, communication skills teaching must seem relevant and not simply 'this is what you need because we're telling you so'.

DISCOVERING LEARNERS' PERCEIVED NEEDS

A starting point for any experiential learning is to discover needs that learners bring with them from their work or experience. What problems and difficulties are they experiencing and what areas would they like help with? What is their previous experience and present level of knowledge and skill? Begin with learners' starting points (where they are), their current problems and needs (their agenda) and where they would like to go (their objectives).

CREATING A SUPPORTIVE CLIMATE

Experiential, problem-based approaches to learning communication skills necessitate the development and maintenance of a supportive climate where learners collaborate rather than compete, where they can gain confidence in themselves, their peers and their facilitators and where they are encouraged to voice their difficulties in a safe and supportive setting.

DEVELOPING APPROPRIATE EXPERIENTIAL MATERIAL

In communication teaching, the material for analysis may be developed by facilitators and course directors (for instance, through simulation or inviting specific patients to participate) or brought by the learners themselves (e.g. in the form of videotapes of their interactions with patients which they bring to the session). When facilitators or course directors are responsible for developing the material, it is important that the setting and case are as close as possible to those which learners will encounter in real life.

TAKING A PROBLEM-BASED APPROACH TO ANALYSING THE CONSULTATION

Whether the consultation is live or on videotape, with real or simulated patients, the problem-based approach starts by asking the learner who has been observed for her agenda: what problems did she experience and what help would she like from the rest of the group? Once this is determined, and if time permits, ask other members of the group if the consultation raised additional issues which they would like to discuss and only then add your own ideas to the agenda if they have not already been raised, especially if they fit in with issues that learners have already identified.

This problem-based, agenda-led approach to consultation analysis reduces defensiveness by ensuring that learners' perceived needs are tackled and that they obtain practical help in overcoming their problems. Practical difficulties that learners are experiencing act as the stimulus for learning. We discuss this approach in detail in Chapter 5.

The balance between self-directed and facilitator-directed learning

But are there not dangers in taking a problem-based approach to communication skills teaching? If we base our approach on discovering and tackling our learners' perceived needs, if we use a learner-centred, self-directed model of learning, are we not overemphasizing the importance of relevance and motivation? What about needs that have simply not yet been perceived by the participants? Do facilitators not have a responsibility to direct learners to their blind spots, to move learners on in their understanding of communication?

In our experience, there is a danger of swinging so far away from teacher-centred instruction towards self-directed learning that learning is unnecessarily compromised. We advocate a collaborative approach to facilitation where self-directed and facilitator-directed learning both play a role. Here, the facilitator is acknowledged to have content expertise in communication skills and balances a learner-centred approach with some direction, introduction to resource material and even occasional brief didactic teaching. Learners are also acknowledged to have experience and expertise which they bring to the group.

Again, the analogy between teaching and the consultation is helpful. We have gradually moved away from a paternalistic doctor-centred approach to the consultation where the control of the interview is entirely in the hands of the doctor and the patient remains a passive contributor. However, consumer-driven consultations where all the power rests in the hands of the patient while the doctor has no say are also often counter-productive, as is the *laissez-faire* approach where essentially no one takes responsibility (Roter and Hall 1992). In the more contemporary patient-centred approach (Stewart *et al.* 1995), it is not that doctors take no role in directing the consultation or that they abstain from offering advice or suggestions; the doctor still helps to provide structure and gives information but as an offer not a *fait accompli*. In the patient-centred consultation, the doctor and patient move toward collaboration and partnership where roles of both doctor and patient remain more flexible .

In teaching, we are saying the same. As collaborative facilitators, we take responsibility for negotiating an agreed structure that helps learners to feel comfortable to contribute. We deliberately encourage a learner-centred approach by basing the discussion on learners' perceived needs and by actively discovering the learners' agenda. But we also contribute our own suggestions and provide appropriately timed information to illuminate and deepen participants' learning.

Problem-based learning does not mean focusing *only* on the learner's perceived problems. It simply means *starting* there as a way into the subject and then assisting learners to take their learning as far as they can. If learners miss an important problem or an opportunity for learning that should not be overlooked, it becomes the facilitator's responsibility to introduce this area into the discussion. Alternatively, it is often appropriate to use learners' issues as a springboard into additional areas of learning. As members of the group, facilitators are free to offer their perspective by raising questions, offering information or role playing a skill. Offered as a definitive solution, facilitator input is counter-productive. But given as an additional alternative to learners' own suggestions which learners have the right to accept or reject as they consider appropriate, such input from facilitators can expand horizons without undermining the problem-centred approach.

Our approach is therefore to incorporate adult learning principles into a structure for learning that balances learner-centred and facilitator-centred activities. Just as in the consultation, an agenda that accommodates both learners' and teachers' needs and perspectives is the most useful.

What place is there for more didactic teaching methods?

Earlier in this chapter, we discussed the evidence that experiential methods of learning are necessary to effect a change in learners' communication skills. This does not mean, however, that *only* experiential methods are of any value and that there is no place for didactic methods in communication skills courses. So what are the advantages of including didactic teaching in the communication skills programme?

Knowledge is important. One of the recurring themes of this book is the need for facilitators to make available to learners the concepts, principles and research evidence that can illuminate experiential learning. Such knowledge allows learners to understand more fully the issues behind communication skills training and the evidence for the value of each skill. Although by themselves, cognitive approaches such as reading, analysing, hypothesizing and classifying do not generate skills, intellectual understanding can augment and guide our use of skills and aid our exploration of attitudes and issues.

Knowledge of the integral relationships between various communication skills is also extremely important. Understanding the logical connection between various skills and how they can be used together in different parts of the consultation can both enhance learning and enable the skills to be used more constructively in the interview. Providing schema that group skills into categories and define their interrelationship enables learners to piece together their learning into a form that they can remember and then use at will. As we have already shown in Chapter 2, learners need to understand the structure and conceptual framework of the consultation to make sense of their learning and to retain it over time.

In Part 2, one topic we explore is how to constructively introduce cognitive material into a predominantly skills-based experiential curriculum while at the same time avoiding the pitfalls of teacher-centred didactic methods.

Part 2

Communication skills teaching and learning in practice

4

Choosing and using appropriate teaching methods

Introduction

In Chapter 3 we presented an overview of how to teach and learn communication in medicine in which we demonstrated:

- the rationale for taking a skills-based approach to doctor–patient communication
- the importance of specific experiential learning methods in communication skills teaching
- the need to incorporate a problem-based approach
- the value of using didactic methods and cognitive materials to complement experiential learning.

But how are these methods used in practice? What didactic and experiential methods are available and what are the advantages and disadvantages of each? How do you extend learners' knowledge and understanding of doctor–patient communication and also maximize their development of skills?

The choice of teaching and learning methods significantly influences the outcomes which communication programmes or individual sessions are likely to achieve. Programme directors and facilitators need to understand the relative merits of each approach and to choose intentionally between them. Since these methods demand active involvement, learners will also benefit from understanding the rationale for their choice. In this chapter, we therefore:

- explore how to choose between the available teaching methods
- examine the use of didactic, knowledge-based teaching methods
- discuss the use and relative merits of the following sources of experiential material:
  - audio and video recordings
  - real patients

– simulated patients
– role play.

Choosing appropriate teaching methods

How do we choose between the various teaching methods that are available for use in the communication curriculum? What can we expect each different method to achieve? Placing the available methods along the following continuum helps guide our decision making:

facilitator centred   learner centred

<--->

didactic –   experiential – leading to   experiential – leading to
'in your head'   deeper discussion/understanding   action/change in behaviour

Methods all along the continuum are useful, none is without merit. Practical considerations such as availability, cost and time constraints all influence the choice of method. But whether a given method is effective depends ultimately on the outcomes you are trying to achieve.

Didactic

The didactic end of the continuum includes lectures, group presentations and reading. Although these methods may be stimulating, they tend not to lead to changes in behaviour or to the development of skills. Such facilitator-centred methods where the learner's role is more passive can stimulate interest, promote thinking, expand understanding and help develop conceptual frameworks, but alone rarely lead to action or sustained change. Didactic methods enable learners to understand what it takes to communicate effectively but do not develop learners' skills or ensure mastery and application in practice.

Experiential methods leading to deeper discussion or understanding

Moving along the continuum towards the middle ground, we find a set of experiential methods which lead toward deeper discussion or understanding but are still removed from changes in behaviour. These methods are, however, more likely to engage the participants and increase the level of response and involvement. Examples include the use of trigger tapes, demonstrations, workshops, discussions and exercises.

Experiential methods leading to action or change in behaviour

Finally, the continuum moves to experiential methods which lead to action or change in behaviour. Here, one learner undertakes an interview while others observe. Learners engage in feedback about the interview, rehearse alternative approaches or specific skills and perhaps try again in part or in full. Performance becomes a significant part of the course content. Experiential methods are more likely to result in experimentation with alternatives, changes in attitude and behaviour, development of skills and strategies (rather than just deepened awareness and understanding) and action. The difference between didactic and experiential methods is the difference between *knowing about* effective communication and *being able* to communicate effectively.

Format: large group, small group, one to one

Didactic learning can occur in many formats including large group, small group, one to one or even solitary settings. For instance, lectures and more interactive demonstrations and exercises can occur in large- or small-group format. Discussion of communication research and theory can take place in one-to-one tutorials, small groups or large groups. Critical reading, assigned literature reviews or project work can be undertaken alone or in small groups. In contrast, experiential, problem-based learning is most effectively performed only in small-group or one-to-one format with expert facilitation.

As communication skills programmes place a heavy emphasis on methods from the right hand side of the continuum, most learning takes place in small-group or one-to-one settings. We discuss the relative merits of small-group versus one-to-one formats in Chapter 5.

The methods continuum is a way to keep the breadth of approaches in mind and assist programme directors and facilitators in choosing appropriate methods for each component of the communication curriculum. The rest of this chapter explores the use of methods from both sides of the continuum in communication skills programmes.

Using methods from the left half of the methods continuum

We have already established that didactic methods are not, by themselves, sufficient to achieve change in learners' behaviour and that experiential methods are required to cement learning from didactic methods into place. However, didactic methods are still important in the communication curriculum:

- cognitive material can motivate learners to 'buy in' to communication skills training. By understanding the problems that occur in medical communication and examining the solutions generated by research to overcome them, by learning about the theory and research behind communication skills and communication skills teaching, learners can comprehend the importance both of studying this subject and of exposing themselves to the potentially uncomfortable process of experiential observation and feedback
- didactic methods can illuminate experiential learning, augmenting learners' understanding of the skills that they are developing and helping them to see the logical connections between them.

Introducing cognitive material into the curriculum

We can introduce cognitive material into communication programmes in a number of ways.

AS AN INTEGRAL PART OF SKILLS-BASED WORK

Cognitive information is best assimilated when learners can:

- discover for themselves a need for information
- actively grapple with the information rather than listen passively to its presentation
- understand the rationale and principles behind the information rather than simply learn it by rote
- understand the logical interconnections and links between different pieces of information
- group together various concepts into memorable categories
- relate the information to its practical application.

In Chapter 5, we introduce *agenda-led, outcome-based analysis*, an approach for teaching and learning communication in which we combine problem-based experiential learning with the appropriately timed introduction of research evidence and other didactic material. This method builds on the above principles by introducing cognitive material at just the point in the learners' experiential explorations when they have generated a need for information and can therefore assimilate it most readily. Any lessons from this information can be immediately tried out in rehearsal to see how they might be of value in practice.

Introducing didactic material is an integral part of the facilitator's responsibilities during experiential sessions. To achieve this, facilitators must have information about communication research and theory at their fingertips. This is a problem for many facilitators who may lack formal training and, despite desires to the contrary, have little time to pursue this information on their own. Our companion book, *Skills for Communicating with Patients*, is designed to help programme directors and facilitators overcome this problem.

AS SEPARATE ACTIVITIES

There is also a definite place for separate, more traditional, cognitive activities including:

- didactic lecture presentations
- assigned literature study
- critical reading of research evidence
- tutorial and discussion groups
- project work
- demonstrations (live or videotape)
- seminars and panels.

Programme directors and facilitators need to consider how to use these various activities within the curriculum. They might, for instance:

- provide a large group lecture or demonstration at the beginning of the course to 'hook' learners
- use discussion groups to augment experiential work throughout the course

- assign literature study or introduce project work or seminar presentations around issues that have surfaced in experiential discussion
- include the use of demonstration or trigger tapes to introduce skills appropriate to a particular section of the consultation
- place large- or small-group didactic sessions strategically throughout the course to summarize learning so far, provide research evidence or introduce a new issue or skills area.

It is important to consider the reasons for exposing learners to each of these activities so that appropriate choices can be made.

Lectures, for instance, are not an effective way of changing behaviour but can act as a hook to learners to enable them to buy into experiential learning. In a compulsory undergraduate communication course, an initial lecture can ease learners into new methods of working by setting the scene and explaining the objectives and teaching methods of the course. In continuing medical education, a lecture can hook learners' interest: it can explain the need for communication training and validate the subject by the presentation of appropriate research evidence. This can act as a spur for practising physicians to attend experiential courses. Lectures can also be used within a course to pull together progress so far and to introduce new areas of learning before moving on to further experiential sessions. Didactic presentations become more effective when they include interaction such as discussion, brainstorming, pairs or small-group exercises within the lecture to stimulate participant involvement in learning.

Critical reading and project work engage learners intellectually and enable them to understand the theoretical and research basis that validates the study of communication skills in medicine, to explore the rationale underlying the use of individual skills and to better understand and participate in their own and their peers' learning of communication skills.

Demonstrations or modelling can act as a valuable introduction to specific communication skills but should not be confused with true experiential training. Demonstration may initiate lively debate about communicating with patients. Trigger tapes of good and bad consulting skills or live demonstrations by an instructor with real or simulated patients may act as a first step in learning communication skills by modelling appropriate behaviours. But, by itself, demonstration only enables learners to know about rather than develop the ability to use communication skills. Learning communication skills requires practice, adaptation and individualization.

We explore the use of demonstrations by the facilitator during experiential learning sessions in Chapter 5. Like lecturing, this technique should be used sparingly as we learn best what we create or re-create for ourselves. Rather than demonstrating a skill and then asking learners to try it out, we prefer to take a problem-based approach that encourages learners to discover appropriate skills for themselves. Only when learners are struggling to generate appropriate skills do we feel it appropriate to make suggestions ourselves from within the group.

Using methods from the right half of the methods continuum

A variety of experiential methods are available which make it possible to observe learners interacting with patients:

- audio and video recordings
- real patients

- simulated patients
- role play.

What are the relative merits of each of these methods?

Audio and video recording

We have already explored the advantages of audio and video review in communication skills teaching programmes in Chapter 3 (Hargie and Morrow 1986; Premi 1991; Beckman and Frankel 1994; Westberg and Jason 1994). Research into communication skills teaching has clearly demonstrated the central importance of the recording and playback of interviews. There is no doubt that video recording represents the gold standard of communication teaching. Although potentially more intrusive and threatening to learners and patients than audiotape, videotape permits a focus on visual aspects of non-verbal behaviour not possible with audiotape, holds the attention of reviewers far better and enables a more detailed analysis of the interview (Kurtz 1975; Westberg and Jason 1994).

PRACTICAL ISSUES IN THE USE OF VIDEO RECORDING

But what are the practical issues involved in using videotape in communication programmes?

1 *Expense*. It is an expensive medium. There is considerable capital outlay required to equip a programme with both the hardware for recording (cameras and microphones) and for playback (television screens and VCRs). Equipment needs to be serviced, maintained and eventually replaced as the march of technology renders the original machinery obsolete. Fortunately, modern, unobtrusive camcorders have become considerably cheaper and more available over recent years.

2 *Technology*. Video technology can interfere with the process of training. Cameras need to be set up, microphones checked and sound levels confirmed prior to recording sessions. Playback equipment needs to be connected and compatible with the recording hardware. Failure of sound or vision in recording or playback can sabotage a session and undermine the confidence of learners and facilitator. To overcome these problems, every effort should be made to simplify the setting up of equipment. The recording equipment should be readily available, preferably permanently *in situ*. In clinical situations or teaching rooms regularly used for video recording, permanently installed camera-mounting brackets and hard-wired microphones help to facilitate recording. Facilitators or other staff members should take responsibility for ensuring the recording equipment is set up and working. Where equipment needs to be moved to the clinical situation, this should be done prior to the recording, without involving patient or learner. Playback equipment should be equally accessible (Kurtz 1975; Westberg and Jason 1994).

3 *Setting*. The setting of experiential learning requires consideration. Some medical schools and teaching hospitals provide the ideal setting of paired observation rooms with one-way mirrors between them. Such rooms can be grouped together in dedicated clinical skills

laboratories and used for many kinds of clinical skills teaching and evaluation. The consultation takes place in one room which is equipped to simulate an examining room or doctor's office with built-in camera and microphone. The small learning group observes, records and sometimes briefly discusses the interview in progress in the second room.

If paired rooms are not possible in your setting, movable dividers can be used to separate observers from doctor and patient. Alternatively, silent observers can sit at some remove and watch the encounter as it is being recorded (the 'fishbowl' technique) or the videotape can be recorded privately without others observing the live interview for use later.

If you are setting up in a clinic, place the equipment as unobtrusively as possible. Fix the camera to permit at least a three-quarter body shot of both doctor and patient together. Unless you can control the camera remotely (and usually even then), resist the temptation to fiddle with different angles or to zoom in for close-ups of facial expression. Such camerawork is distracting and of little benefit for video review. During physical examination of patients which requires the removal of clothing, ensure that the camera is positioned so the examination cannot be seen or block the lens so that only sound recording continues during the examination.

4 *Time*. Using video and audio during teaching sessions takes time. Replaying the whole tape or even sections of the recording adds considerably to the length of the teaching session. Handling videotape efficiently requires expertise on the part of the facilitator, particularly if selected skills and behaviours are sought as the session progresses. It is helpful if group members note down specific tape times or counter numbers as they watch interviews so that short sections can be found and replayed during feedback or so that learners can refer to those specific moments when reviewing the tape later.

5 *Apprehension*. The use of videotape can add to the fear and apprehension of observation (Hargie and Morrow 1986). If being observed and receiving feedback is unsettling, it can be even worse enduring a live camera in the corner of a room and being forced to watch your behaviour in glorious Technicolor. The very advantages of using recording and playback (self-assessment, learner involvement, objectivity, accuracy, specificity of feedback, description and microanalysis of behaviour) can all cause discomfiture to learners (Beckman and Frankel 1994). This approach needs careful handling and we explore in depth how to achieve this in Chapters 5 and 6.

Despite these potential difficulties, video recording remains a most valuable tool for communication skills programmes. Rather than holding back the use of video work, these issues need overcoming as the benefits to learners and teachers are so significant. The immediate benefits to learners are clear from the research that we have described in Chapter 3. But longer term benefits also accrue. Learners can keep a record of the encounter and review the teaching session later to reinforce learning. The programme director can also keep a record, perhaps developing a bank of interviews to assist in future teaching or for use in preparing trigger tapes (brief recordings used as triggers for discussion and role play). Recordings can also assist in research and development of the course as well as in student evaluation, as we see in Chapter 8. Additional permission of patients and learners is *mandatory* for any use of their tapes in research or education that extends beyond the immediate use for which the original consent was obtained.

Real patients

The use of real patients in the communication skills curriculum can take several forms.

PRE-RECORDED VIDEOTAPES OF REAL CONSULTATIONS

A common experiential method used in residency training and CME is the video recording of real consultations that have taken place within the learner's own practice. This has become the standard approach to communication skills training in British postgraduate general practice and has much to recommend it. As discussed earlier, it is important that experiential material explores situations that are as close to reality as possible. What could be more real than a true consultation, videotaped in the doctor's workplace? Participants can bring interviews that they have found to be difficult and can ask the group for help with specific issues.

In addition to problem-based work, videotapes of real consultations can be used in two other ways:

1 learners can video all their consultations over a period of time to ensure that certain issues which have proven difficult in the past (such as explaining the use of steroid inhalers to re-luctant parents of asthmatic children) are captured on tape for later review and discussion
2 once confidence in videotape analysis and a supportive environment for learning have been established, learners can video a whole clinic session and select consultations for analysis at random. This produces a more accurate picture of learners' performance.

Bringing pre-recorded videos to the communication course in this way has its drawbacks. The patient cannot personally provide feedback to the doctor on their performance and is also not available for further rehearsal: alternative methods using role play have to be employed. We know that recording and observation is not enough by itself; further rehearsal is also neces-sary for new behaviours to be incorporated into the learner's repertoire. We therefore need to engineer rehearsal in all experiential sessions that employ recordings. This is relatively easy with simulated patients – the group can watch the interaction between 'patient' and doctor as it occurs, the video record can be used immediately afterwards during feedback and further rehearsal with the actor can take place. Rehearsal can, however, be more difficult when using pre-recorded videos of real patients who are not present at the time of the teaching session. Here it is important for one member of the group to watch the recording from the patient's perspective and be prepared to role play the patient during feedback and rehearsal. We describe this technique more fully in Chapter 5.

LIVE INTERVIEWS OF PATIENTS BROUGHT TO THE COMMUNICATION UNIT

An alternative way of using real patients is to bring them to the communication course to be interviewed expressly for the purpose of helping learners. For example, facilitators who are practising doctors can invite selected patients to participate in the programme. Or if the learn-ing facility is attached to a hospital, arrangements can be made with nursing staff for in-patients to participate.

Using real patients in this way can be of considerable value. For instance, at the beginning of the undergraduate communication curriculum, learners are eager to see real patients and value the opportunity to practise with patients in the safety of the communication unit. Immediate feedback from the patient can be extremely valuable to learners – they can discover if a line of questioning was handled sensitively from the patient's perspective or if the patient wanted more information than the learner had assumed (Kent *et al.* 1981). Unfortunately, patients are sometimes so supportive to learners that they find it difficult to make constructive criticisms!

Using real patients in this way poses other difficulties.

1 *Rehearsal limitations.* Although trying out alternatives is possible, repeated rehearsal can be difficult for real patients. Real patients often have trouble both picking up the thread of the consultation at the point where a particular problem appeared and behaving differently in each rehearsal: they are not actors. These difficulties increase in parallel with the complexity of the situation. Rehearsing how to take a history efficiently with a real patient is relatively easy; asking a patient to allow several students to try different techniques to elicit hidden depression is clearly a different matter.

2 *Restricted types of patients.* Only certain types of patients will be able to participate; for example, retired people who are free during the day. Patients seen tend to be those with chronic conditions in general practice or patients in hospital who are now stable – they are clearly a selected group.

3 *Realism.* The medium itself greatly influences the interviews that are observed. Much of the realism of a true interview is negated by the way in which the interview has to be engineered. Because it is a repeat interview, most patients will not present the symptoms or their concerns in the same way as when they saw the doctor initially. The patient may no longer have an acute problem and may only be able to tell the doctor of problems they had in the past. Much of the emotional climate will have been ameliorated by what has happened to them since their initial interview. We can hardly expect a patient to replay going through the process of anger at the medical profession, experiencing severe pain or receiving bad news. Therefore we cannot expect to teach how to cope with such demanding situations with this approach.

4 *Consent.* Consent is, of course, a major issue in any situation in medical education where real patients are invited to help learners. This is particularly true when recordings are made. Truly informed consent is necessary and patients must be given a genuine opportunity both to refuse to participate and also to change their minds after the consultation (Southgate 1993; GMC 1995). Safeguards such as informing the patient that no intimate examinations will be recorded, that minors must be accompanied by an adult, that the tape will only be seen by doctors and those responsible for their education, and that the tapes will be kept secure and erased after a certain period of time need to be clear on the consent form. The patient must sign before and after the consultation to give fully informed consent.

There is conflicting evidence about the degree to which patients object to their consultations being videoed. Five studies from British general practice show the following results. Martin and Martin (1984) found a low refusal rate of 16%. The figure was even lower if the doctor personally asked the patient to participate. Servant and Matheson (1986), however, found an unusually low figure of only 6% agreement to participate in patients who had to actively 'opt in', that is, positively volunteer to have their consultations videotaped and Myers (1983) found that the longer the time patients had to consider video recording, the more likely they were to refuse. Bain and Mackay (1993) found that just under half of patients attending surgeries and given questionnaires said that they would feel under pressure to participate and three-quarters said that they would feel uncomfortable. Campbell *et al.* (1995*b*), in a study of matched patients from two practices, found that there was no difference in satisfaction ratings between those who had their consultations videotaped and those who did not.

There is clearly some concern that patients may feel coerced into having their consultations recorded and might agree to do so to 'please the doctor' or ensure that their care is not compromised. This is an important ethical matter which we encourage you to look into carefully in cooperation with appropriate governing bodies, professional organizations and your institutions' ethics and legal advisors.

Asking receptionists rather than the doctor to obtain consent from patients reduces the likelihood of coercion. However, we have found that receptionists need to be trained for this task to ensure that patients are given a genuine choice; they must make it clear that the doctor will not mind if the patient prefers not to be videotaped.

Simulated patients*

Simulated patients have been used successfully in communication teaching, evaluation and research since their first introduction in the 1960s (Barrows and Abrahamson 1964; Helfer and Levin 1967; Jason *et al.* 1971; Werner and Schneider 1974; Maguire 1976; Stillman *et al.* 1976, 1977, 1990*a*; Callaway *et al.* 1977; Kahn *et al.* 1979; Kurtz 1989; Anderson *et al.* 1994; Hoppe 1995; Kurtz and Heaton 1995). Also known as professional, programmed or standardized patients (especially when trained to 'perform' a role consistently for evaluation and research purposes), simulated patients portray live interactive simulations of specific medical problems and communication challenges to order. Initially, real patients were used to produce standardized presentations of illnesses they themselves had previously experienced (Barrows and Abrahamson 1964; Helfer *et al.* 1975*b*; Stillman *et al.* 1976). Simulated patients are now more commonly either professional or amateur actors or trained members of the community without formal acting background who portray roles from outside their own experience (Barrows 1987).

Simulated patients provide opportunities for learners to experiment and learn in a protected, safe environment, without the possibility of harming real patients, yet in as close an approximation to reality as possible. The use of simulated patients has been shown to be acceptable to learners and faculty and to be effective, reliable and valid as a method of instruction and evaluation (Fraser *et al.* 1994; Vu and Barrows 1994; Hoppe 1995; Bingham *et al.* 1996). Simulated patients are realistic patient substitutes; research demonstrates that students, residents and practising physicians cannot distinguish between real and well-trained simulated patients (Burrie *et al.* 1976; Sanson-Fisher and Poole 1980; Norman *et al.* 1986; Pringle and Stewart-Evans 1990; Rethans *et al.* 1991; Saebo *et al.* 1995). The availability of simulated patients offers particularly rich opportunities to communication skills programmes.

* We are indebted to Brian Gromoff, Director, Simulated Patient Program, University of Calgary for his suggestions and assistance, which we have relied on throughout this discussion of simulated patients.

ADVANTAGES OF SIMULATED PATIENTS

1 *Rehearsal.* Simulated patients provide ideal opportunities for rehearsal during feedback sessions. Here is the ultimate offer to learners: feel free to experiment and to rehearse skills over and over again – do what you can hardly ever do with real patients in the outside world and say out loud 'That didn't work the way I wanted it to, let me try it again differently'! Simulated patients are willing for learners to make mistakes and to provide multiple opportunities for trial and error so that learners can practise skills in safety without any adverse consequences of 'botching' an attempt at a new skill. Of course, this is only possible if the actor is present at the time of the group's discussion of the consultation. It is not available if the interview is recorded before the group meets and the simulated patient is not present when the tape is reviewed.

Simulated patients can be used very flexibly within the communication unit. They can participate with or without the addition of video recording in the setting of purpose-built, paired rooms with built-in, one-way mirrors as described earlier in this chapter. Or they can simply join a group of learners and practise interviewing skills without any of the paraphernalia of the modern skills laboratory. Here, either the actor and learner can sit apart from the rest of the group while they watch in silence (the 'fishbowl' technique) or the actor can become part of the group itself with everyone in the group participating in interviewing and rehearsals.

2 *Improvisation.* Simulated patients are able to replay parts or the whole of an interview, to re-enter the consultation at any point, reacting appropriately and differently each time as participants try varying approaches. These improvisational qualities are very important as they enable the value of different behaviours to be seen in action. They also enable the learner to stop the consultation at any point to discuss what is happening; the actor can remain in suspended animation and can then pick up the consultation whenever the learner or another member of the group is ready to continue. As we have described, it is unfair to expect real patients to rehearse complex or difficult situations repeatedly and be able to change their behaviour in relation to the doctor's skills. However, actors have the great advantage of being trained to immediately re-enter situations as if they had never been there before and give a fresh performance each time. Their flexibility is invaluable.

3 *Standardization.* Simulated patients can also provide standardization, i.e. reproducibility of roles. Different learners can face the same challenge on different days. Learners can learn from how their peers cope with identical situations. Facilitators and programme directors can work out criteria for evaluation and feedback in advance and even try out communication challenges for themselves. Standardization of simulated patient roles has enabled great strides to be made in the assessment of clinical competence and in the research of communication skills.

4 *Customization.* The use of simulated patients allows the interview to be customized to a particular learner's level and tailored to their needs. Simulated patient cases can be varied so that once core skills have been mastered, the degree of challenge can be increased.

5 *Specific communication issues and difficult situations.* Simulated patients are able to portray cases that demonstrate particularly difficult situations and are therefore ideal for helping with

dedicated sessions on specific issues. Programme directors can plan ahead and guarantee that the curriculum will cover situations such as breaking bad news, cultural issues, addiction or anger which might well not arise opportunistically if we rely solely on situations that learners experience during the time-span of the communication course. Asking real rather than simulated patients to come to the communication unit to replay many times their own difficult or emotionally charged experiences is clearly inappropriate. Using simulated patients overcomes such problems.

6 *Availability*. Simulated patients can be available whenever required without disturbing real patients. A bank of specific cases can be developed and made available to the communication or other faculty at a moment's notice. They can simulate out-patient, house call, emergency or bedside consultations. Being freed from the constraints of patient availability allows the communication programme much greater choice as to when sessions can take place.

7 *Time efficiency*. The use of simulated patients is time efficient: particular skills can be isolated and practised without observing an entire interview. It is possible to run through many stages of the progression of an illness in quick succession so that learners can follow through the consequences of communication skills in action. In one day, students can experience the events that in real life might take several weeks. An example of this is used in the integrative course of the undergraduate programme of the University of Calgary (see Chapter 8) when a patient with ischaemic heart disease is followed through from out-patients, to admission, to intensive care, to sudden death, while simultaneously his wife is also interviewed at admission, at the time of breaking bad news and when threatening legal action.

8 *Feedback*. An important advantage of involving simulated patients in communication skills training lies in their ability to provide feedback to learners and give insights from the lay perspective. A group of medically trained learners and facilitators can so easily forget to include the patient's perspective in their discussion. Indeed, it could be said that medical training makes it impossible for doctors to see issues entirely from a patient's point of view without their accumulated medical experience providing an impenetrable fog that obscures the lay perspective. Simulated patients, however, can explain how they feel as the patient, providing feedback that would otherwise remain unavailable (Jason *et al.* 1971; Whitehouse *et al.* 1984; Barrows 1987).

9 *Facilitation, instruction and evaluation*. Increasingly, simulated patients have also been trained to act as facilitators, instructors and evaluators, further extending their role in the communication programme. In these circumstances, they are often called patient instructors (Helfer *et al.* 1975*a*; Carrol *et al.* 1981; Stillman *et al.* 1983; Levenkron *et al.* 1987). Here, they are not just giving feedback in role as the patient but are also commenting out of role on the interview skills used by the learner in much the same way as a facilitator. Simulated patients' feedback can be used in both formative (Stillman *et al.* 1976, 1977, 1990*a,b*; van der Vleuten and Swanson 1990; Sharp *et al.* 1996) and summative assessment of learners' skills (Stillman and Swanson 1987; Langsley 1991; Grand 'Maison *et al.* 1992; Vu *et al.* 1992; Klass 1994; Pololi 1995) and can play an important part in research into communication skills and communication skills teaching (Burri *et al.* 1976; Roter *et al.* 1987; Roter and Hall 1987; Monahan *et al.* 1988; Hoppe *et al.* 1990).

CHALLENGES IN THE USE OF SIMULATED PATIENTS

Several practical issues influence the use of simulated patients in communication programmes.

1 *Expense*. Simulated patients are expensive and unlike the capital costs involved in purchasing video equipment, this cost is recurring. Actors rightly require payment for both acting and preparation time and we should not undervalue their time financially. You may be lucky and find retired or 'resting' actors who provide their time voluntarily but this cannot be relied upon.

Actors are often eager to participate in communication programmes. Their reasons include the opportunity to improve their improvisational skills, to learn about portrayal of a variety of characters and problems, to learn feedback skills and to enjoy the benefits of expert coaching and additional, if intermittent, employment. Schools of acting often provide student actors who are more than willing to help free of charge, but, as we shall see, there are major issues here for actor training that probably outweigh financial considerations.

The personnel costs of faculty members, trainers and educators in developing cases, selecting and training simulated patients and devising evaluations as well as the costs of providing space, equipment and administrative support also need to be considered (King *et al.* 1994).

2 *Selection*. The selection process for simulated patients is important, both before and during training. Simulated patients may be either professional or amateur actors, drama students or trained members of the community without a formal acting background. It is wise to exclude candidates who have negative attitudes towards the medical profession. Simulators must come across as having a genuine desire to help rather than a propensity for putting doctors or learners down. Many people have experienced poor communication with health professionals at first hand. This in itself can be helpful, providing simulated patients with valuable insights into the issues and skills under discussion. It is more the degree of anger, defensiveness and hostility that needs to be considered when selecting potential simulators. Another potential problem is the individual with unresolved issues that relate to a particular case. Such personal agendas are usually inappropriate in simulation and can cause difficulties for both simulator and learner.

Drama students can prove to be excellent simulated patients. However, students sometimes lack the maturity to understand their role in aiding learners rather than scoring points off them and, depending on their level of expertise, they may overact. They also move on each year which means that the effort expended in training has to be repeated annually and a bank of simulated patients is never developed.

Recruiting members of the community without an acting background via word of mouth or advertisement can also be worthwhile; they can come from existing patient populations, community organizations, disease-focused foundations, amateur theatre groups or simply be interested members of the public. Useful attributes to look for are an interest in helping doctors to learn, an ability not just to memorize a role but to adapt flexibly to different interviewer styles, the ability to express emotions verbally and non-verbally, reliability, physical stamina and emotional stability (King *et al.* 1994; Pololi 1995).

Unless individuals are previously known to the trainers, each candidate must be screened carefully through an application and interview process; special care should be taken in screening individuals from the community at large for their protection as well as your own. Obtaining a candidate's personal medical history is an important part of the process.

3 *Training*. Simulated patients also require training (King *et al.* 1994). It is vital for the success of the programme that simulators are trained to depict accurately the behaviour of patients in various settings, to portray specific roles, to understand the objectives and methods of the communication skills programme and to give well-intentioned and constructive feedback (Barrows 1987). For instance, it may not be intuitive to a simulator that patients often give covert rather than overt clues to their underlying need to ask questions or that they shy away in the first instance from doctors' direct questions about their ideas or concerns. Simulators need their own experiential training in all these areas: observation, feedback and rehearsal are just as important for actors as for learners. Regular monitoring of roles with feedback and refinement are necessary.

Simulators also need to be in tune with the objectives of the communication skills programme: they need to understand what communication training in medicine is hoping to achieve and to comprehend the difficulties that learners might have in buying into a programme which is attempting to change their behaviour. If simulators will be asked to give feedback, they need to understand the principles of giving well-intentioned, constructive and non-judgemental feedback that will support learners and enable them to change.

They also need some understanding of the 'what' of communication skills, especially if they are to give feedback not just in role about how the patient is feeling, but also out of role about communication skills *per se*. In role, the feelings expressed are those of an individual patient; out of role, the simulator may be acting more as a group member or facilitator. Simulators must therefore consider their comments made out of role more carefully. Actors can make excellent facilitators and provide valuable 'out of role' feedback but if course organizers expect actors to adopt this responsibility effectively, they must provide them with a degree of training similar to that given to other facilitators.

Before moving on to train for a particular role, simulated patients require a brief, general orientation to the communication programme, to the ethos and teaching methods of the unit and to any responsibilities they may have in teaching or evaluating learners.

In Calgary, the training process for a particular role involves the simulated patient studying the written case they are to portray and discussing it with a trainer. Rehearsal comes next, with a trainer or sometimes other actors experienced in the programme in the role of doctor. Trainer, simulated patient, sometimes the physician who wrote the case and, more rarely, the person upon whom the case is based then discuss misperceptions, answer questions and offer suggestions for more realistic portrayal. Rashid *et al.* (1994) and Thew and Worrall (in press) have described an approach to training simulated patients in which a videotape of the original consultation on which the case has been based is used.

For more complex cases or when standardization is important (e.g. if the actor is participating in certifying examinations) additional preparation might include small-group learning where actors portraying the same or different roles watch each other's performances and then participate in experiential feedback sessions. Videotapes may be made of these rehearsals and of performances with learners for later review either independently or with the trainer or a small group of other actors. The simulation can be 'tested' for authenticity by having the physician who wrote the case or a clinician who has not seen it conduct the interview. If physical findings or specific communication challenges are a part of the simulation, these are taught (if possible) and tested along with the history.

Once a case is 'in performance', trainers ask those facilitating the learning for feedback and perform checks to make sure that the patient maintains consistently accurate portrayals. It is all too easy to start mixing cases up or inadvertently change or forget crucial elements; retraining is often required. Depending on the complexity of the case, training in one role requires two to eight hours, with further time required if the simulator is to act as a patient-instructor and provide oral or written feedback (King *et al.* 1994; Pololi 1995).

4 *Hidden agendas.* Although most learners comment on how realistic and useful simulated patients are, learners occasionally feel that they are being 'set up' by the facilitator and actor. Learners sometimes think there are hidden aspects of the role that they are being asked to discover, akin to peeling away the skins of an onion until the real flesh is found. As only the actor and facilitator know the details of the patient's story in advance, it can appear that they are deliberately planning to trip up the learner. This suspicion can be reduced by introducing the actors (or at least the fact that actors will be used and why) to the group early on. Of course, some aspects of the case are there to challenge the learner's communication skills but it is important that learners see this as a chance to practise skills rather than as a 'set up'. Using real cases with events that happened in actual practice as the basis for the simulation rather than making cases up also helps to resolve this problem.

5 *Programme director's time.* The last practical issue to consider is the time it takes to develop cases, to recruit, train and follow up simulated patients and to organize them to be available at appropriate times. In a large programme it can become impractical for the programme directors to do all of this themselves. Appointing staff specifically dedicated to this task may become necessary.

In Calgary, the appointment of a director of the Faculty of Medicine's simulated patient programme (from a background of acting, directing, producing and teaching drama) led to a significant and wide-ranging expansion of the simulated patient programme throughout the faculty, in both undergraduate and postgraduate programmes and into both coursework and evaluations. While the programme originated in the communication unit, a bank of standardized patients and cases was developed that could be called upon by programme directors of any course whenever required. New cases could be developed on request with an expertise and knowledge of the process of role development and training that would otherwise not be available to the various programme directors throughout the medical school. This enabled the use of simulated patients to spread beyond the communication unit and led to greater acceptance and integration of communication skills teaching throughout the faculty as a whole.

DEVELOPING SIMULATED PATIENT CASES

Simulations are more realistic if based on real patient cases, with name and details altered to protect anonymity. The original history may be adapted to make it more appropriate for particular learners by increasing or decreasing the complexity of the problem. A simulated patient case is often devised by a case development team that might consist of the doctor who originally saw the patient, the programme organizers, the simulated patient trainer, educators involved in the evaluation programme and other health professionals. (For a good review of the literature see King *et al.* 1994.)

Although different approaches are possible, the method of case development that we favour is the production of a written case. Relevant details are organized under the headings of the traditional medical history (presenting problems, history of present illness, past history, family and social history, etc.). The write-up usually begins with a brief summary of the case and its context (both place, such as emergency room, ward, doctor's office, and circumstances, such as first or follow-up visit, previous relationship with the doctor). The write-up also includes relevant details about the patient's personality, affect and relationships. Brief directions concerning aspects of the patient's communication are included such as how much information the patient originally offered or items that the real patient mentioned only when asked explicitly. If they are part of the case, communication challenges are clearly stated and often contain some specific wording that the simulator is asked to incorporate. Details of history or demography that are not explicitly written can be filled in by the actors from their own personal history if they wish, but care must be taken not to introduce 'red herrings' that demand attention but have nothing to do with the case. The case usually includes a sentence or two providing information about the setting or patient that learners would have before meeting a real patient. This is read to all learners just before the consultation with the simulated patient begins.

For cases which integrate communication and physical examination, we include appropriate physical findings and results of laboratory or other investigations. Supporting materials may take the form of slides or computerized visuals of actual X-rays or scans presented without the real patient's name and used with permission. For some cases we provide these data for both original and follow-up visits, adding complications that arose over a period of time but which students can experience through simulation in the course of an afternoon.

These 'scripts' contain information; they do not contain dialogue apart from occasional suggestions for phrasing (usually to do with specific communication challenges). We supply these write-ups to the facilitators as well as the simulated patients so that facilitators have a written document clarifying the details the learner might be expected to elicit and can explain the context before learners meet the patient. Some facilitators prefer to involve themselves as learners or as physicians seeing the patient for the first time as they observe – they look at a new case write-up only after they work on the case in collaboration with their learners.

Role play

Role play is another valuable method that we use to advantage in the communication curriculum (Bird and Cohen-Cole 1983; Simpson 1985; Maguire and Faulkner 1988b; Coonar 1991; Koh et al. 1991; Mansfield 1991; Cohen-Cole et al. 1995). We have already discussed how role play is an integral part of all experiential methods involving rehearsal: group members are encouraged to adopt the doctor's role during the analysis of the consultation to practise and rehearse skills. We have also seen how in consultations that have been recorded earlier and in which the real or simulated patient is not available to take part in the discussion of the interview, we invite a participant to adopt the role of the patient to facilitate feedback and rehearsal.

Here we discuss a specific form of role play where one learner becomes the patient for an entire interview. The learner role-playing the patient may be given a particular role to play (e.g. through a printed 'script' which describes the details) or alternatively 'creates' the role herself based on a medical problem she has experienced personally or seen as a doctor. A second learner (who does not know the case) plays the doctor. Afterwards, the group analyses the interview as usual. There are clear advantages to this method:

- it is cheap – in fact, free!
- little, if any, training is required
- it is always available – it can be done whenever the programme director wishes without planning and without much organization. Tapes do not have to be prepared in advance or actors trained and booked
- it allows some learners to adopt the patient role, a significant learning experience in itself
- role play enables easy, repetitive practice of specific interviewing skills with ready access to instant observation, feedback and re-rehearsal
- it can be used during any teaching session, both inside and outside the communication curriculum, whenever facilitators or learners wish to practise communication skills relevant to a specific topic. A group which is familiar with role play can slip in and out of this method with ease.

Role play is useful in various circumstances.

1 *Difficult cases*. Role play can be used in an impromptu fashion to illustrate difficult cases that learners have experienced in their work and that they bring to the learning group. Reverse role play is particularly valuable here: the doctor who has experienced a difficulty takes the part of a patient with whom he had a problem while another participant plays the doctor. Alternative skills can be demonstrated while at the same time the initial doctor can gain valuable insights by experiencing the patient's feelings at first hand.

2 *Problem scenarios*. Learners can be asked to develop their own role plays to demonstrate the specific problem or area of the interview which is the focus of the current teaching session. These role plays can be based on scenarios that they themselves have experienced in real life as students, doctors or as patients.

3 *Specific communication issues*. Scripts of patient and doctor roles can be developed by the facilitators prior to the session so that a particular issue can be explored and discussed in detail. One approach here is for two participants to portray patient and doctor and for the subsequent interview to be videotaped and analysed in the same way as it would be with a simulated patient. Alternatively, role plays can be performed simultaneously by dividing the group into pairs of doctor and patient or trios of doctor, patient and observer. Each unit performs and analyses the interview without videotape. Having one person as an observer helps the remaining pair to take the exercise seriously and provides valuable, descriptive feedback during the analysis. This technique can be used in large as well as small groups; everyone can be working on their communication skills at once.

4 *Trigger tapes*. After they have watched prepared trigger tapes, learners can be invited to adopt the roles of both patient and doctor on the tape. This is of particular value when it has proved difficult to obtain experiential material and the only material available is prepared tapes not involving the group participants. As discussed earlier, just watching and analysing trigger tapes can enable learners to understand communication skills intellectually and increase the response from learners but, by itself, is unlikely to change behaviour or increase

skills. However, the addition of participant role play can convert the use of trigger tapes into an experiential method that does enhance skill development. The tape serves as a launching pad for rehearsal and role play of new skills that learners suggest for dealing with problems that they identify on the tape.

DISADVANTAGES OF ROLE PLAY

The disadvantages of using role play relate to the degree of difficulty participants may have in adopting roles. Participants are not actors and can find it difficult at first to role play without self-consciousness, especially if they already have a relationship with the other participant. In particular, they may find it difficult to shed their medical knowledge and react as if they were a patient without the background expertise and experience which in real life the learners have. It is easier for learners to role play a problem they have experienced themselves (with enough personal details changed to protect privacy) or to portray real people such as a patient the role player has seen in real life or on video. It is much more difficult for learners to adopt a role from scratch: most learners find it difficult to improvise a history as they go unless a reasonably detailed background is provided. It can often feel artificial to both 'doctor' and 'patient' if the 'patient' is not able to sink herself into the proposed role. This artificiality is the most common criticism of role play. Care is therefore necessary in preparing learners for role play, especially for the 'patient' who may need help entering the role play situation.

The problem of 'unreality' in experiential learning

All the experiential methods that we have discussed are valuable in providing opportunity for observation, feedback and practice. Unfortunately, all are likely to be criticized by learners (and sometimes faculty) as being 'unreal'. Working with video recordings of real patients is unreal because the technology and consent forms can affect the interview. Working with simulated patients is not the same as the real thing. Conducting an interview with a friend role-playing the patient is not equivalent to interacting with a real patient.

These difficulties should always be acknowledged – after all, they are true! Any method of observation is bound to interfere with the process of the interview. But they are still the best methods that we have for helping learners to develop skills. Although we should accept learners' reservations that they are not showing themselves to their best advantage, we should remain aware that the underlying tension that produces such statements is often not concern about the accuracy of the situation but anxiety about being observed and criticized in the first place. This natural defensiveness and concern about competence needs to be accepted and understood.

A valuable way of defusing this performance anxiety is to agree that the situation is unreal but to make the point that unfortunately reality does not allow you to observe and then experiment: here is an opportunity to make mistakes in safety, to be immune from causing harm and to replay interviews time and time again, something that never happens in real life. And anyway, things do not go as planned in real life either – we are often performing below our best because of interruptions, disruptive thoughts or tiredness. We have to find a way to cope in many situations where the conditions are not perfect.

5

Running a session: analysis and feedback in experiential teaching sessions

Introduction

We turn our attention now to strategies for running individual small group or one-to-one experiential sessions. We have already seen that communication teaching and learning needs to:

- be skills based
- use observation, feedback and rehearsal in active small-group or one-to-one learning
- place considerable emphasis on experiential methods such as video review of consultations with real or simulated patients or role play
- take a problem-based, experiential approach to learning
- incorporate cognitive material and attitudinal learning.

So how do you put all this into practice? How do you run a session combining all the necessary elements? How do you structure experiential sessions to maximize both learning and safety? How do you combine experiential and didactic learning? And how should facilitators and learners phrase feedback so that defensiveness is minimized and learning encouraged?

In this chapter, we look at a specific approach to facilitating communication skills sessions that enables us to meet these challenges. We concentrate on two separate but overlapping themes:

1 how to structure analysis and feedback in communication skills teaching sessions:
   - why is there a need to organize feedback and learning in communication skills teaching?
   - conventional rules of feedback: strengths and weaknesses

- an alternative approach: *agenda-led, outcome-based analysis* of the consultation
- how to use agenda-led, outcome-based analysis in practice

2 how to phrase feedback in communication skills teaching sessions:
  - the principles of constructive feedback
  - SET–GO descriptive feedback.

Structuring analysis and feedback in communication skills teaching sessions

Why is there a need to organize feedback and learning in communication skills teaching?

We know that didactic teaching methods are not by themselves successful in teaching communication skills as they do little to change learners' behaviour. Yet didactic teaching does have certain characteristics which teachers in many fields find appealing:

- it is safe, at the expense of being unchallenging to a mostly passive learner
- it is structured: the teacher has a plan which is set out at the beginning and progresses until the end. The teacher is in control and can impart considerable information in a short period of time
- the subject matter covered is clearly apparent: a series of lectures can cover a syllabus with some confidence.

In contrast, although experiential skills-based learning is essential to produce change in learners' communication skills, it introduces several difficulties which must be overcome if we are to create successful communication programmes:

- **it is potentially unsafe:** the more challenging a method is to learners, the more risk they take. Exposing yourself to criticism is never easy and in the wrong environment, negative or unsupportive comments from the leader or other learners can block potential learning. Learning communication skills is not the same as learning other skills: because communication is closely bound to self-concept and self-esteem, learners can perceive suggestions for change as a threat to their personality. Extra efforts are necessary to ensure a supportive, safe environment
- **it is less structured:** it is a more 'messy' environment to work in than didactic teaching with less apparent structure. The more learners become involved in collaborative learning, the more difficult it is to structure the session to ensure useful learning for all. It is so easy for experiential learning groups to make inefficient use of time or to reach vague and non-productive end-points
- **by nature, opportunistic and random:** facilitators can never entirely predetermine the skills that will be covered in any one session. The focus will vary depending on what happens to take place in the observed interview, the flow of the session and the particular needs of the learners. Facilitators may have difficulty ensuring that the curriculum of skills is covered and learners may have problems piecing together the random parts of the puzzle that slowly emerge.

The challenge is therefore to minimize the difficulties associated with experiential teaching while at the same time maximizing the valuable learning opportunities. Communication skills teachers have developed several approaches for structuring analysis and feedback in experiential sessions to achieve both safety and learning (Riccardi and Kurtz 1983; Pendleton *et al.* 1984; Gask *et al.* 1991; Lipkin *et al.* 1995; Silverman *et al.* 1996b). Here, we contrast an established method of organizing feedback with an alternative approach – *agenda-led, outcome-based analysis* of the consultation.

Conventional rules of feedback

We first describe a method for structuring feedback that has been used extensively in communication skills teaching over the last decade. This approach was formalized in relation to feedback in medical education by Pendleton *et al.* in 1984 and is often referred to as 'Pendleton's rules'. The rules have become part of many published approaches to the teaching of communication skills in medicine (Pendleton *et al.* 1984; McAvoy 1988; Cohen-Cole 1991; Gask *et al.* 1991).

These rules of feedback were introduced primarily to provide safety in the analysis of the consultation. Pendleton and his co-workers observed the tendency for feedback in medical education to emphasize learners' omissions and failures and to omit supportive and constructive advice about how to change. Learners often perceived observation to be a destructive experience that did not induce a willingness to learn. Pendleton's team therefore recommended ground rules to reduce this potential danger. They specified an order to feedback which insisted on good points first and ensured that an overall balance to feedback was achieved.

These ground rules have been variously interpreted, not always in the form that Pendleton *et al.* originally intended. The following, however, is one interpretation in widespread use:

- briefly clarify matters of fact
- the learner being observed first says what was done well, and how
- the rest of the group, or the facilitator alone in one-to-one work, then comments on what was done well, and how
- the learner then says what could be done differently, and how
- the rest of the group, or the facilitator alone in one-to-one work, then says what could be done differently, and how.

The educational principles underlying these rules are:

- *positive first for safety*. Pendleton *et al.* suggested that 'learners' strengths should be discussed at length before any suggestions are made', that 'deposits are made before withdrawals'. This was proposed in order to prevent negative criticism producing a spiral of attacking and defending. Insisting on discussing strengths first was intended to engender a safer and more supportive climate. Positive reinforcement of strengths also occurs
- *self-assessment first*. Learners should have the opportunity to make comments about their own interview first. For the learner, it is much more helpful to be able to own a difficulty for oneself than to be criticized about something before having a chance to mention it: much defensiveness can be reduced. For the facilitator, understanding the learner's awareness of problems via their own self-assessment is important 'diagnostic' information. There is a considerable difference between the learner who can appreciate that a difficulty has occurred and the learner who has not recognized that there is a problem

- *recommendations not criticisms.* The conventional rules stress the importance of going beyond saying that something was not done well. For learning to occur, recommendations have to be made about how the difficulty might be put right. The rules therefore suggest that feedback only be given when a suggestion for change can be provided – not just 'what was wrong' but 'what could have been done differently and how'.

The development of these rules was an important contribution to addressing the difficulties with feedback apparent in the early days of consultation analysis. Their introduction was helpful in preventing learners from receiving only negative criticism. But as medical educators have gained increasing experience in this complex field, it has become apparent that there are difficulties within the rules that can limit the method's learning potential. Their central tenets – balanced feedback, self-assessment and the provision of suggestions for change – remain as vital today as when they were first introduced. However, it is the rules' insistence on a strict order to feedback that can create problems without necessarily providing the safety that was their primary intention.

WHAT ARE THE POTENTIAL DIFFICULTIES OF THE RULES?

1 *The artificiality of separation of good points and problem areas, of learner and group.* In order to ensure safety, the rules insist on a strict ordering of feedback, with good points having to be made before difficulties are discussed and with the learner having to make comments before observers are allowed to contribute. The facilitator acts as a policeman, directing who contributes and when comments can be made. This creates an artificiality about the feedback process. It frustrates discussion by preventing points from being made when they are thought of or when they are most appropriate. Considerable time can separate comments about specific areas of the consultation which can then become difficult to remember or relate to each other.

The learner may wish to say:

'I thought I introduced myself well but I could have just checked who the person was who came in to the room with the patient'
or
'I see what you mean about my questions being very thorough but I felt that if only I'd used more open questions, I could have discovered so much more'.

Adhering to the conventional rules, facilitators have to intervene with:

'Hold on, we're only on good points at the moment.'

The rules seem to suggest that ensuring safety through the strict observance of the order of contribution is of more importance than enabling an interactive discussion. Yet often participants comment that this approach is overprotective, that constructive criticism is inhibited. If we are trying to promote an interactive approach to the consultation itself, should we be attempting to prevent it in our communication teaching? The emphasis on ever-present danger necessitating restrictive rules can, paradoxically, feel very unsafe.

2 *Evaluative phrasing of feedback.* Despite their aim of preventing destructive feedback from having an adverse effect on the learner, feedback given under the conventional rules can still

come across to learners as evaluative and judgemental. By contrasting 'what was done well' with 'what could be done differently', the conventional rules inadvertently set a judgemental tone for the feedback that follows. The rules attempt to ameliorate this perception of evaluation by suggesting that feedback on 'good points' is followed by 'recommendations rather than criticisms'. While this helps, in learners' minds 'what could be done differently' is still often seen as a thin disguise for 'what was done poorly', especially as it is so directly contrasted with 'what was done well'. The learner may therefore perceive the initial positive feedback as patronizing or insincere (as sugar-coating) and be bracing herself for the 'hit' she thinks is sure to come.

As we shall see later in this chapter, evaluative feedback tends to create defensiveness, reducing safety and inhibiting learning. For learning to occur, we need to move our language away from the evaluative framework of 'good and bad' and find alternative ways of phrasing feedback that learners can more readily accept.

3 *The learner's agenda is discovered late in the feedback process.* The rules do not discover the learner's agenda until late in the proceedings. Insisting on good points first prevents the learner from having an early opportunity to mention particular areas that she perceives to have been difficult and with which she would appreciate help from the rest of the group. Paradoxically, this approach may make the person receiving feedback more anxious; she may not be able to take in the initial comments about her good skills as she is worried about how her problems are being assessed by others. Uncertainty may lead to anxiety which may block her ability to hear comments about her good skills and so diminish the potential learning from this very important aspect of feedback.

4 *Inefficient use of time.* Too often the group spends a disproportionate amount of time on the 'good' with too little left for constructive help with the difficulties of the consultation. It is tempting to try to be as supportive as possible by teasing out all the good points in the consultation, especially if there are difficult areas to discuss later.

The process can be repetitious: separation of feedback is cumbersome, leading to one area being covered several times in the feedback process. Because all of the learner's good points in the whole of the consultation are produced first, followed by all the group's good points, then all the learner's suggestions and then all the group's suggestions, the consultation is continually criss-crossed from one end to the other. It becomes difficult to concentrate specifically on one section of the consultation and consider it in any detail.

Agenda-led, outcome-based analysis of the consultation

We now describe agenda-led, outcome-based analysis, an alternative method for analysing consultations which maximizes learning and safety in experiential sessions (Silverman *et al.* 1996*b*). It overcomes the disadvantages of the conventional rules that we have outlined above while building on the rules' strengths of preventing unbalanced negative criticism and promoting self-assessment. In addition to changing the way feedback is structured, this approach encourages a delicate mix of problem-based experiential learning, centred on the learner's agenda, with the appropriately timed introduction of concepts, principles, research evidence and wider discussion. The potentially random and unstructured nature of experiential communication skills teaching is overcome so that learners can more readily develop an evolving, structured understanding of the communication curriculum. The approach that we describe here works in both small-group and one-to-one teaching. It is equally appropriate for the analysis of live interviews (i.e. the interview is conducted and possibly videotaped as other learners and/or the facilitator observe – feedback follows immediately) or pre-recorded videotaped interviews (i.e. the interview is conducted and videotaped away from other learners or the facilitator – observers later watch the videotape and provide feedback) (Riccardi and Kurtz 1983; Kurtz 1989; Heaton and Kurtz 1992b).

The principles of agenda-led, outcome-based analysis (Box 5.1)

START WITH THE LEARNER'S AGENDA

The key to this method of analysis is that it is agenda led: the discussion starts by asking what problems the learner experienced in the interview and what help she would like from the rest of the group. What are the advantages of this approach?

- It allows a problem area to be discovered and acknowledged early on, preventing anxiety and uncertainty from blocking the learner's ability to appreciate feedback.
- It is more efficient and structured as the group homes in on a particular problem and attempts to solve it together.
- A specific section of the consultation can be addressed and analysed in depth.

Starting with the learner's agenda is contrary to the conventional rules' suggestion that good points should come first. But, in fact, starting with the learner's agenda is often safer and more supportive than starting with a self-assessment of strengths. Because the learner is identifying a problem area for herself and inviting the other members of the group to help, defensiveness is reduced. Simply acknowledging her difficulties allows the learner to become more relaxed and able to hear the impressions of others. Damaging feedback is rarely a problem: the group generates a supportive climate from the outset and willingly takes to its task of helping the learner to work out alternative strategies. The key step here is the request for assistance: feedback to help solve a difficulty is openly invited.

As we shall see, balanced feedback is still essential but follows on from this initial step of discovering the learner's agenda. Often, facilitators and learners feel that insisting on good points first can feel strained and artificial; they feel that learners have difficulty finding any good points to recognize in their performance. But, in fact, learners may be simply blocked by their own unstated agenda which is still uppermost in their mind and needs to be acknowledged first. Just as in consultations with patients, we benefit from discovering and accepting learners' thoughts and feelings rather than blocking their expression.

The important step here is providing the opportunity for the learner to start with her agenda if she has one and if she wishes to share it with the group. Sometimes, the learner does not have a specific agenda or is unable to articulate it initially. She may simply ask for feedback first from the group. This is fine – it is not so much that the analysis has to start with a detailed agenda from the learner but that she is given the chance to offload her problem areas first if she wishes.

Box 5.1   Principles of agenda-led, outcome-based analysis

- **Start with the learner's agenda**. Ask what problems the learner experienced and what help he would like from the rest of the group.
- **Look at the outcomes learner and patient are trying to achieve**. Thinking about where you are aiming and how you might get there encourages problem solving – effectiveness in communication is always dependent on what you are trying to achieve.
- **Encourage self-assessment and self-problem solving first**. Allow the learner space to make suggestions before the group shares its ideas.
- **Involve the whole group in problem solving**. Encourage the group to work together to generate solutions not only to help the learner but also to help themselves in similar situations.
- **Use descriptive feedback to encourage a non-judgemental approach**. Descriptive feedback ensures that non-judgemental and specific comments are made and prevents vague generalization.
- **Provide balanced feedback**. Encourage all group members to provide a balance in feedback of what worked well and what did not work so well, thus supporting each other and maximizing learning – we learn as much by analysing why something works as why it does not.
- **Make offers and suggestions; generate alternatives**. Make suggestions rather than prescriptive comments and reflect them back to the learner for consideration; think in terms of alternative approaches.
- **Rehearse suggestions**. Try out alternative phrasing and practise suggestions by role play – when learning any skill, observation, feedback *and* rehearsal are required to effect change.
- **Be well intentioned, valuing and supportive**. It is the group's responsibility to be respectful and sensitive to each other.
- **Value the interview as a gift of raw material for the group**. The interview provides the raw material around which the whole group can explore communication problems and issues – group members can learn as much as the learner being observed who should not be the constant centre of attention. All group members have a responsibility to make and rehearse suggestions.
- **Opportunistically introduce concepts, principles, research evidence and wider discussion**. Offer to introduce concepts, principles, research evidence and wider discussion at opportune moments to illuminate learning for the group as a whole.
- **Structure and summarize learning so that a constructive end-point is reached**. Use the *Calgary–Cambridge observation guide* to ensure that learners piece together the individual skills that have arisen into an overall conceptual framework to structure and summarize the session.

LOOK AT THE OUTCOMES LEARNER AND PATIENT ARE TRYING TO ACHIEVE

One of the principles of communication that we outlined in Chapter 2 is that effective communication requires planning and thinking in terms of outcome. The skills that you deploy depend very much on what you want to achieve. Consider the patient who is angry. If you wish to end the consultation quickly and escape from a potentially dangerous situation you will behave in one way; if you wish to understand the underlying reasons for that anger and rebuild a relationship, entirely different skills are required.

Therefore, after discovering the learner's agenda, the next step is to ask what outcomes the learner would like to have achieved. Discuss where the learner would like to get to before looking at the skills that might be effective in achieving that goal. We often also ask the group to consider what outcomes the patient might have in mind – that too influences what is most effective in a given situation.

There are two advantages to taking an outcome-based approach. Firstly, it encourages learner-centred problem solving. By asking the paired questions 'Where do the patient and I want to go to?' and 'How might we get there?', the learner and the group become actively involved in setting their own objectives and in discovering appropriate skills to satisfy their own and their patient's needs. Secondly, the outcome-based method encourages a non-judgemental approach. It ceases to be a matter of whether something was intrinsically good or bad and becomes an issue of whether what was done was effective in achieving a particular objective ('what seemed to work' and 'what didn't seem to work' in getting to your chosen outcome). Skills then do not have to assume a moral tag; they are simply useful in different circumstances to achieve different ends.

This is not just semantics: the outcome-based approach is a major factor in reducing defensiveness and facilitating learning. Without an intended outcome around which to base discussion, you are forced to be judgemental, to say something was implicitly good or bad. This carries the suggestion that there is a definite right or wrong approach that the giver of feedback is party to. At the very least, feedback becomes subjective, a personal judgement of little constructive use to the learner who might simply disagree.

The outcome-based approach enables the learner to state what she would like to have achieved in the interview and then receive feedback about approaches and skills that would help her achieve her own objectives. She is not so much being judged as being helped to attain her own goals, and by examining what worked and what did not in achieving this task, the language of feedback naturally moves from an evaluative to a non-evaluative mode.

ENCOURAGE SELF-ASSESSMENT AND SELF-PROBLEM SOLVING FIRST

The conventional rules emphasize the importance of always allowing the learner space to comment first. This initial self-assessment, so helpful to both learner and facilitator alike, is also central to our method.

However, we also promote the related concept of self-problem solving by involving the learner as early as possible when the group or facilitator provides feedback. In the conventional rules, when it is the group's turn to make comments, group members are asked to provide alternative suggestions when they give feedback about 'what could have been done differently and how'. This means that the learner being observed is left out of the discussion until after an alternative strategy has been presented. The learner becomes a passive recipient of others' ideas.

In contrast, we encourage the group not to provide solutions immediately, but instead to simply describe what they see and reflect this back to the learner:

'At 0:45, I could see that you were looking through the notes to find out what you did last time and the patient then became rather hesitant. What do you think, Sue?'
'Yes, I think you're right. Perhaps I could have put the notes down and just maintained eye contact in those first few minutes.'

This gives the learner an opportunity to acknowledge what happened and problem solve herself before the group makes suggestions. The group can then provide further help and a supportive interaction is achieved. Both self-assessment and self-problem solving reduce the potential for defensiveness that occurs when learners receive suggestions on areas that they are quite able to work through for themselves.

INVOLVE THE WHOLE GROUP IN PROBLEM SOLVING

We have seen how starting with the learner's agenda and using an outcome-based approach encourages problem solving. Once problems are identified and outcomes determined, the whole group can make suggestions as equals about how to solve the dilemma. It becomes a matter of approaching the problem rather than the learner's performance. Of course, the learner should have the opportunity to go first but the key to this approach is to involve the learner and the rest of the group together. The group can then work to generate solutions not only to help the learner but also to help themselves in similar situations which they will undoubtedly face in the future or have already done in the past. This creates an equality between the learner and the group and prevents the learner being the constant centre of attention.

USE DESCRIPTIVE FEEDBACK TO ENCOURAGE A NON-JUDGEMENTAL APPROACH

Descriptive feedback is a very simple method of providing non-judgemental, specific, behavioural and well-intentioned feedback. Later in this chapter we explore how to phrase feedback by describing what is seen and heard without initial interpretation or evaluation.

PROVIDE BALANCED FEEDBACK

The conventional rules correctly insist on balanced feedback, not only to support the learner but also to maximize learning: we learn as much by analysing why something works as why it does not.

But is it necessary to focus so strictly on good points first before making any recommendations? We have found that if effort is expended to provide a supportive environment, if an agenda-led, outcome-based approach is used in the analysis of the consultation, if the group is working together in joint problem solving, then the order of feedback is not of such crucial importance. Responsibility ultimately rests on the facilitator to make sure that balanced feedback occurs by the end of the session but he can be much more flexible about the order in which this feedback is given and can abandon the artificiality of insisting that all good points appear before any difficulties can be discussed. Comments about what worked well and what did not in a particular part of the consultation can be given together, thus opening the way for useful interaction between the learner and the group: learning can be maximized. This approach requires the facilitator to monitor the climate of the group and the position of the learner throughout the session: in certain situations, if defensiveness is already in the air, it may be more important to start with some areas that worked well. But mostly, if the group is working well together, achieving a balance by the end is all that is necessary.

Such supportiveness may not come naturally to learners brought up in the competitive world of traditional medical education. For this approach to work, considerable effort needs to be expended to create a supportive environment, stifle defensiveness and encourage collaborative learning. Rather than imposing rules that keep learners in check, we prefer to discuss our approach openly with the group first, to explore the potential gains and difficulties, promote a supportive climate and encourage a problem-based approach. We invest our efforts in carefully observing balance and support, stepping in if necessary to redirect, checking with learners as to their needs and providing structure to the learning session to help everyone achieve their ends. This method clearly requires considerable skill and expertise from the facilitator. Yet once the ideas of agenda-led, outcome-based, problem-orientated analysis are established, the problem of safety is largely not an issue.

WORK TOGETHER TO PROVIDE A SUPPORTIVE ENVIRONMENT

In collaborative learning, it is the responsibility of each member of the group to help and support their colleagues. Agenda-led, outcome-based analysis embodies two aspects of this behaviour:

1 *make offers, suggestions and alternatives.* Learners are encouraged to make suggestions rather than prescriptive comments, to provide offers for the learner to consider. Tentativeness rather than certainty, open-mindedness rather than dogmatism, the valuing of alternative viewpoints rather than the giving of prescriptive advice: these approaches aid a problem-solving approach yet they are not the usual stock-in-trade of medical parlance! Again, this models the very skills that we are trying to promote in the medical interview: a collaborative and equal rather than a paternalistic and superior approach to working with patients

2 *be well intentioned, valuing and supportive.* It is the group's responsibility to be respectful and sensitive to each other in order to maximize learning.

REHEARSE SUGGESTIONS

It is essential to rehearse, practise and explore the value of suggestions, not just by discussing them but by trying them out through the use of role play. Rehearsal or practice is the key to learning any skill, the third part of 'observation, feedback and rehearsal'. Rehearsal allows learners to try out suggestions in practice to see if they are advantageous, to experiment with exact phrasing and to transform ideas into practice. Rehearsal leads on to further feedback on the rehearsal itself, to further new suggestions and more rehearsal. It allows learners to experiment with different ideas in safety and to practise for difficult situations in the future.

USE THE INTERVIEW AS A GIFT OF RAW MATERIAL FOR THE GROUP

Approaches which gear analysis and feedback primarily towards the benefit of the person being observed rather than the group as a whole paradoxically increase pressure on the individual and induce defensiveness. We can be so centred on the participant that our attempts to protect her and ensure that feedback is relevant to her needs only serve to put her more 'on the spot' and actually feed the feeling of discomfort.

In contrast, agenda-led outcome-based analysis is deliberately intended to be a group activity. The participant offers a gift to the group which everyone in the group is privileged to be able to experience and from which all can learn. The interview is viewed as a resource to improve skills – a springboard for further learning – rather than as material for evaluation. Learning becomes a group activity between equals that does not just revolve around the participant in the interview. The observed interview provides the raw material which the group can use to explore communication skills and issues: group members learn as much as the learner participating in the interview. Everyone makes and rehearses suggestions. As other participants try out alternatives and receive feedback, the learner is no longer the entire centre of attention.

We clearly have two concurrent aims in our teaching sessions on communication skills:

1 to help the learner being observed with his agenda by involving the whole group, *including himself*, in problem solving to the benefit of all
2 to generalize away from the specific interview in question to look at particular communication skills and issues and to structure overall learning.

This intention to use the interview as 'raw material' or a 'springboard' for further learning needs to be discussed with the group early on and become part of the group contract.

OPPORTUNISTICALLY INTRODUCE CONCEPTS, PRINCIPLES, RESEARCH EVIDENCE AND WIDER DISCUSSION

At appropriate points and with the permission of the group, the facilitator can generalize away from the interview in question to:

- explain principles of communication
- present (or ask others in the group to present) research evidence
- clarify specific skills or concepts through demonstration (modelling), discussion, brainstorming, exercises, etc.
- focus attention on specific areas of the interview.

The facilitator can pick up on the group's current discussion and offer any of these approaches to help learners explore a skill or topic further. After such teaching, the facilitator can return to the learner in the initial interview to see if the discussion has been helpful.

This kind of teaching needs to be introduced at points where it will most help learners and complement their self-exploration; in other words, in response to problems and issues that learners have already identified. It is a mistake to think that all the work of the group must be experiential without any input from the leader. Facilitators have knowledge that can illuminate the working of the group. Sharing such knowledge is valuable as long as the facilitator encourages equality of contribution, does not hog the floor, keeps inputs brief, avoids pre-empting ideas learners can come up with on their own and remains a learner within the group. Learners can then decide on the value of the leader's contribution and accept or reject its usefulness as they wish.

Using the interview in this way has important advantages. Firstly, the learner visibly relaxes as the spotlight is removed and the learner has an opportunity to sit back and contemplate. The group becomes much more involved in the learning process and is placed in a position of equality with the learner receiving the feedback. Secondly, it enables learners to see the broader picture and to structure and pull together their learning so that a constructive end-point is reached. We have already mentioned how experiential learning is potentially unstructured and random – here is one way to counter the problem by a subtle mix of experiential learning, group work and brief didactic teaching.

STRUCTURE AND SUMMARIZE LEARNING SO THAT LEARNERS DEVELOP AN EVOLVING AND SYSTEMATIC UNDERSTANDING OF THE COMMUNICATION CURRICULUM

Communication skills teaching and learning naturally focuses on the present agenda and problems of the learner. Learning occurs opportunistically in the areas that happen to arise during the interview that is observed. How then can we ensure that learners piece together the apparently randomly arising individual skills into any sort of overall conceptual framework? How can learners keep an overview of what has or has not been covered so far in any session or over the course as a whole? How can facilitators structure and pull together the specific skills that are identified as the session proceeds to prevent them from looking like a disorganized bag of tricks?

As a first stop, communication training programmes need to define the content of the curriculum. In Chapter 2 we presented the *Calgary–Cambridge observation guide* which both describes a comprehensive set of individual skills that make up the focus of a suggested curriculum for medical communication skills training programmes and also provides a framework for structuring these skills that mirrors the consultation.

The use of the Calgary–Cambridge observation guide in the everyday teaching situation to structure learning over time. Having defined what we are teaching, we need to enable learners to piece together the skills that arise at random in their learning. We do this by using the guide during everyday teaching sessions as a concise, accessible summary of communication skills for facilitators and students alike. This provides both an *aide-mémoire* that learners and facilitators can easily refer to during sessions and a method of countering the random nature of experiential learning. It gives a framework within which to place the individual skills and build up an overall schema. By listing the skills in the form of observable behaviours shown to be useful at different points in the consultation, the guide allows appropriate areas to be highlighted and practised as they arise.

We encourage learners to keep the guide in front of them during observation and feedback and either to write on it directly or refer to it as they write notes on a separate sheet of paper. The guide is not intended to be used as a check-list with items ticked off as the means of giving feedback. Check-lists foster a pass/fail attitude that stifles rather than promotes learning. Instead, participants and facilitators are encouraged to write detailed, specific and descriptive comments on the form to guide their discussions. We have produced versions of the guide that offer space for recording comments within the structured sections of the guide (*see* Appendix 2). This encourages observers to consider where in a consultation the interviewer is at any one time and where he should be aiming for. The guide is a tool for self and peer assessment and can provide a record of others' comments for the learner to take away.

The use of the guide as a method of summarizing the session. A particularly effective use of the guide is as an aid to summarizing and recording the learning that has occurred by the end of a session so that learners can conceptualize their learning more precisely. This is an important final step in agenda-led, outcome-based analysis. The facilitator (or another group member) can reiterate the skills that have been discussed and explain how they fit into the structure of the consultation. She can provide an overview of what has and has not been covered in the particular consultation or teaching session. Learners can later use the guides as an *aide-mémoire* in the consulting room to allow them to practise the skills that have been identified. The facilitator can start the next session by enquiring how the participants have progressed with these skills since they last met.

Here then is a way of structuring learning over time so that maximum use can be made of the experiential methods so essential to communication skills programmes. As we see in Chapter 8, communication courses need to be designed in 'helical' fashion; one-off courses are of little value. The communication curriculum needs to run throughout medical education as a whole, with built-in repetition, refinement and increasing complexity. The guide offers a way of piecing together the skills that occur randomly throughout this helical curriculum so that they are used to their greatest advantage.

How does agenda-led, outcome-based analysis work in practice?

So how do you run an experiential communication skills teaching session in practice that enables the principles that we have outlined above to be put into action? The conventional rules are attractive in their brevity – a few brief lines encapsulate a highly memorable, albeit rigid, structure to the analysis of the consultation. We find it more difficult to be as concise in our own recommendations as our sessions are more complex and follow less of a pre-determined path, relying more on facilitator skill to keep the session flowing, balanced and on course.

Our approach is to first allow time to discuss the principles of agenda-led, outcome-based analysis with learners and then to work within the framework given in Box 5.2 to achieve these principles in practice. Please note that the order is flexible and all participants are encouraged to contribute at all times. Feedback is an interaction and not a direct transmission process; it is dynamic and helical – an exact parallel to the consultation. The process is malleable – do not take the structure as set in stone!

Certain suggestions outlined in Box 5.2 require further amplification.

SHARING WHAT THE LEARNER KNEW BEFORE THE CONSULTATION

Before watching the interview, the group needs to understand the context, to be in a similar position to the learner before he started the consultation. This is particularly important with pre-recorded interviews between participants and real patients. Ask the learner doing the

---

Box 5.2   Agenda-led, outcome-based analysis in practice

Prior to watching the interview

- If using a pre-recorded tape, ask the learner showing the tape to set the scene, describe his prior knowledge of the patient and list the extenuating circumstances! We should know exactly what the learner knew and was feeling when the patient entered the room and no more. If watching a live interview, the group should be given the same information about context as the learner.
- Instruct the group to write down specific words and actions as an aid to descriptive feedback; if using video, jot down exact times or counter numbers.
- Ask one member of the group to watch as if the patient and to role play the patient afterwards to enable rehearsal. This is not necessary if a real or simulated patient is present who can help with further rehearsal during feedback.

After watching the interview

- Allow the group several minutes to collect their thoughts and identify the one or two most important points they would like to bring up in feedback, making sure to provide a balance between what worked and what was problematical.
- Facilitator to consider where to place feedback on what worked well.
- Acknowledge any feelings of the learner who has been observed.

Start with the learner who has been observed

- 'What areas do you want to highlight as being problems for you? Tell us your agenda.' Write up or summarize agenda items.
- 'What help would you like from the rest of the group?'
- 'What outcome would you like to achieve from the feedback session?'
- Facilitator to consider whether to add in his own or the group's agenda here.
- Negotiate with the learner the best way to look at the interview – choose which area to focus on or replay first.
- Invite the learner to start off looking at his own agenda by reflecting on relevant parts of the interview and asking him to use descriptive feedback to say what worked well and what did not work so well – replay relevant parts if working from videotape.
- Elicit thoughts and feelings of learner and patient, including the outcomes they wanted to achieve at various points in the interview.
- Rehearse with one of the group role playing the patient or with the simulated or real patient if present.
- Encourage offers and suggestions from the rest of the group and further rehearsal.
- Obtain feedback from the patient.

Box 5.2 Continued

To the group as a whole

- Summarize progress so far and ask the group for their help; prompt with SET–GO feedback (see later in this chapter).
- Rehearse suggestions.
- Add in facilitator's ideas and thoughts.
- Appropriately introduce theory, research and wider discussion.
- Clarify with the learner that his agenda has been covered.
- Ask the group for any agendas of their own that have not been covered already.
- Be very careful to balance what worked well and what did not work so well by the end.

Ending

- Ask what everyone has learned (one thing to take away) and whether the feedback was useful and felt acceptable.
- Pull together and reflect on the 'what': the structure and skills related to the guide.

---

interview to say what he knew about the patient before the interview started, whether this was a new or review appointment, what he had read in the notes before speaking with the patient, whether he was running late, etc. For pre-recorded interviews it is helpful if the group is not told what happens in the consultation or information that the learner gleaned afterwards so that the group can experience the consultation from the same perspective as the learner. If watching a live interview, the group should be given the same information and instructions as the learner.

Making notes

It is very important for the learner and the group to make notes as they watch the consultation as an aid to giving feedback. Our instructions to the group are to write down as the consultation proceeds the actual words and actions that they hear and see without necessarily attempting any initial analysis. This approach encourages descriptive feedback. If videotape is being used, we also ask them to note the time of key points on the tape so that we can more easily find and replay those areas. It can also be helpful to ask one observer to record details of the content of the history or of explanation and planning so that in discussion the content of the interview can be related to communication process skills.

The importance of the 'patient role'

We cannot overstress the importance of the 'patient role' in feedback and rehearsal. This is easily achieved when working with simulated patients. They can provide immediate feedback of their own unique experience as the patient and replay parts of the interview so that learners can try out suggestions and alternatives. Real patients can also join the group for the beginning of the feedback session to give their impressions, perceptions and feelings.

However, when working with video review of pre-recorded, real consultations, rehearsal and feedback can prove more difficult as the real patient is not available during the feedback session. We can overcome this problem by inviting one member of the group to watch the interview as if they were the patient on screen, to be prepared to give feedback as the patient afterwards and to role play the patient whenever suggestions are rehearsed. This method brings several advantages:

- it provides a way to rehearse new skills and alternatives
- the participant playing the patient will have observed the consultation from the patient's perspective and, to a degree, will have become patient rather than doctor centred. Although this lay perspective is bound to be contaminated by medical training, the presence of some-one in the patient role alters the dynamic of the group. The discussion loses that adversarial feeling of doctors talking about patients in a 'them and us' way so recognizable to anyone who has witnessed doctors or students having a coffee break. The 'patient's presence' reduces posturing and allows us to listen to the patient.

Taking turns role playing the patient gives learners an insight that is denied them when working with simulated patients. Experiencing the patient's perspective is highly educational for any learner. We learn so much from our own illnesses about the doctor–patient relationship – here is another method of experiencing this without actually having to be ill!

HOW TO ENSURE A BALANCE IN FEEDBACK

Facilitators new to this method of structuring a session often comment about the apparent difficulty of ensuring that 'what worked well' is highlighted as much as 'what did not work as well'. Looking at the consultation from an agenda-led, problem-based perspective is likely to emphasize the difficulties that the learner experienced. If you start with problems, perhaps it is all too easy to miss out on successes. Certainly, this approach does not have a defined place for the 'positive': discretion and responsibility are left in the hands of the facilitator to ensure that a balance is eventually achieved.

There are several possibilities for introducing 'what worked well' into the discussion. The choice of where to place it will depend on how the group is working, the level of support demonstrated by group members, the degree of anxiety apparent from the learner doing the consultation and the level of trust that has been established. Here are some examples.

- One method is to discover the learner's agenda first and then reflect on or replay the relevant-portion of the interview. Invite the learner to start by saying what worked well and then continue with what difficulties occurred. This is rather like applying the conventional rules to a small chunk of the consultation but there are big differences. Firstly, agenda items have already been divulged and acknowledged – the learner has already asked for help with his problem from the group and is therefore more able to listen to comments about what worked well. Secondly, looking at a small chunk of the consultation prevents the consultation being criss-crossed from one end to the other. As feedback is restricted to one area of the interview, what worked well and what did not are not separated by large tracts of time and the group can take a problem-based approach to one section of the consultation.
- When the group is well established and working supportively, a frequently used method is simply to trust the group and 'go with the flow'. Start with the learner's agenda, reflect on

or replay the appropriate portion of the interview and let the learner start with his own suggestions for approaching the difficulty. Let the flow of descriptive feedback and rehearsal of suggestions continue and, in most circumstances, the feedback from learner and group will include enough comments on what worked well to balance the analysis of the problem areas. The facilitator should ensure that what worked well is analysed in depth so that learning can occur here too. If positive feedback has not surfaced during the feedback session, the facilitator should ensure that enough time is left towards the end. She can openly ask the group for their feedback on what worked well by stating that the group is in danger of not giving balanced feedback and starting by providing an example herself.

- Sometimes, the learner is keen to move straight into his own suggestions for change. It is important to flow with this and offer him plenty of opportunity for role playing the scenario differently. Feedback can then be given on the role play: much of it will focus on what worked well in the new approach. This may be enough: the learner has provided his own self-assessment, solved his own problem, rehearsed his suggestion and received further feedback – little else is required. In the rare situation where little went well in the original consultation and few helpful skills have been demonstrated, it is perhaps more honest to give balanced feedback on the replay than make up half-truths about the original. Ask the learner to role play suggestions for alternatives and invite discussions about these new efforts and skills; otherwise, forced 'positive' feedback can feel like dishonesty or collusion.

- Looking at the section of the interview leading up to the point at which the learner perceives a difficulty can be helpful. Often it is an appropriate use of skills that has allowed the learner to get to the point where things have gone awry. For example, the patient may have dropped several cues about his concerns which the learner did not pick up; but they would not have surfaced at all if the learner had not employed skills of facilitation and non-verbal communication. Although the learner's agenda is the missed clues, it would be instructive to start by looking at what worked well to allow the interviewer to get to that very point. This ensures balanced feedback.

- If the group is not yet settled or if the learner doing the interview is inexperienced or uncomfortable, it is possible to say immediately after the agenda has been discovered: *'George, now that you've told us your agenda, would you prefer to spend a few minutes looking at what worked well overall before we look at the agenda items in depth?'*. Because George has already asked the group for help with his problems, he will be able to gain benefit from this positive feedback. It does not have to be exhaustive. A brief time spent here will help to flag up to the group the extra need for balance as the analysis moves ahead.

- Another method is for the leader to add 'what worked well' into the agenda-setting process at the very beginning: *'OK, so that's what you would like us to concentrate on. I'd also like to suggest that we look at some of the things that worked well for you so that we can all learn from that too – there were certain things that I think would be very valuable to highlight – what do you think – which should we take first?'*. Note the parallel to agenda setting in the consultation.

ACKNOWLEDGING THE LEARNER'S FEELINGS

Before setting the agenda, it is important to ascertain and acknowledge the learner's feelings. Just as in the consultation itself, it is vital to develop an early awareness of the emotional climate. It is important to discover if the learner is upset, embarrassed or distressed and to accept and support his feelings. This does not mean that we should jump to the defence of what happened in the interview and attempt to rescue the learner by reassuring him that it was perfectly all right. There are more appropriate ways to provide support and ameliorate learners' distress than by offering premature, global and possibly inaccurate feedback.

Imagine the learner who starts by saying:

'That was terrible. I handled it really badly. I was in such a rush that I talked all over him.'

Responding with the alternative global judgement:

'I don't agree. It was fine – you found out all you needed to know – what more can you do when you're behind time?'

does little more than devalue the learner's self-assessment and provide false reassurance – no doubt he does have a point even if his distress may have exaggerated the situation. Instead of positive feedback at this point, it is more appropriate to accept the learner's feelings, using acknowledgement and empathy to provide support:

'I can see that you are not happy about the interview. I guess that time pressure is a problem for all of us and that we've all been in similar positions before' – then check out with the group to get their support – *'I'm sure that it would be helpful for us all to work out some strategies to deal with this issue'*

or to provide support and feedback about something else rather than on the skills in question:

'That was exactly my agenda for this interview as well – recognizing the problem is half the battle, so well done. How can we best help you with it? Do you already have some ideas of your own?'

SETTING THE AGENDA

As discussed earlier in this chapter, the learner should be given the opportunity to present his problem areas first. We spend some time establishing the participant's agenda prior to looking at the specifics of the interview. We ask what problems the learner experienced and what help he would like from the rest of the group. These responses can be written on a flip chart so that the group can refer to them periodically.

In most situations, the learner's agenda and the facilitator's coincide sufficiently for the facilitator to see how he might incorporate any feedback that he considers important into the ensuing discussion. Sometimes, however, the learner misses an important area that the facilitator feels should not be overlooked. Either the facilitator can wait until the detailed exploration of the participant's agenda has been completed before introducing a new agenda item or he can add it into the agenda-setting process just as one might in the consultation:

'So, you'd like to explore the difficulty you experienced at the beginning of the interview in establishing why she came today and also how to explain the risks of hypertension to a worried patient. I wonder if we could also spend a little time looking at how to gauge what information the patient might want from us? I think it might be an interesting area to explore in this interview as well.'

Which approach the facilitator uses depends on the maturity of the group and the participant's level of defensiveness. If the learner is already showing signs of defensiveness, it might be best to stick to the learner's agenda at first and gauge the advisability of proceeding into more threatening areas as the discussion proceeds. If the group is working well together, it is appropriate to be quite open about other possible agenda items by inviting all members of the group to suggest areas they would also like to explore.

LOOKING AT INTENDED OUTCOMES

Exploring outcomes is important, first during agenda setting with regard to what the learner wants from the feedback session, and again at specific points during the interview in relation to what both learner and patient wanted to achieve in the consultation. Sometimes, the outcome wanted by the learner is at odds with that of the patient or the facilitator and maybe the rest of the group. Sharing these different outcomes allows a non-judgemental exploration of skills: we can look at the skills that we might use with different outcomes in mind rather than implying that a particular use of skills is intrinsically right or wrong.

Learner: *'What I wanted to do was not make too much of an issue of her blood pressure and just reassure her that it only needed checking in a month. I didn't want to go into the risks associated with hypertension at this stage; that would only worry her unnecessarily.'*

Facilitator: *'What would other people have wanted to achieve at this point? How about the patient – what did she want?'* or *'Yes, I can appreciate that. I think I'd have liked to find out whether she was already worried and what she already knew about high blood pressure – I wonder if there is a way of gauging that? I guess we could look at both approaches, how to reassure and how to discover if the patient was already worried and see what skills we might need with each.'*

MAKING USE OF THE VIDEO (OR AUDIO) TAPE

Replay the tape frequently, particularly when it is difficult to remember exactly what happened during the interview. During feedback sessions, replaying the appropriate portion of the tape enables feedback to be more specific and concrete and allows the 'patient' to enter into role plays more readily. In cases where feedback focuses on live interviews that are taped as the group watches, encourage the learner to watch the entire tape after the session. Ask the group to jot down specific comments and suggestions on the guide so the learner can take the notes and refer to them as he reviews the tape later.

ENCOURAGING THE EXPRESSION OF THOUGHTS AND FEELINGS

Encourage the exploration of the learner's and the group's thoughts and feelings to allow an understanding of how our perceptual processes influence (help or hinder) our interaction with patients.

REHEARSAL

Encourage learners to try out suggestions as soon as possible in the feedback process in order to shift away from theoretical discussions that remain 'in the head' and move towards the reality of carrying out suggestions in practice. It is easy otherwise to stay safely in the realms of generalization, theory, conjecture and assumption rather than move towards the specific identification and practice of usable skills:

'Try putting some of your ideas into action. Go back to where the patient said "I'm really concerned this might be cancer ..." and take it from there.'

'So you think an open-ended question might have worked better there. How would you phrase it? Assume I'm the patient, ask me ... Anyone else want to try another alternative?'

INVOLVING THE GROUP

As the agenda-led method of analysing the interview starts with the learner who has performed the interview, the discussion in the initial stages tends to be restricted to a duo of learner and facilitator as together they set the agenda and negotiate how to address the problems identified. However, it is important to bring other learners into the discussion as early as possible or they may be relegated to the role of silent observers.

There is a tension in the early stages of the session between the needs of the individual and the group. For instance, if the learner is immediately able to identify possible solutions to his own problems, give him the opportunity to role play the scenario differently himself, even though this will keep the participants out of the discussion even longer. However, as soon as it is possible, invite group members to make suggestions and role play their offers. Once others have contributed to rehearsal, the nature of the group will move from learning for the learner to learning for all members of the group. It is then the facilitator's responsibility to encourage everyone to contribute, to trust the group and let it have its head for a while before coming back in to summarize or redirect.

GENERALIZING AWAY TO INTRODUCE RESEARCH AND THEORY OR ADD DEPTH TO DISCUSSION

As we have already said, the timely introduction of cognitive material and wider discussion into experiential work are important responsibilities for communication skills facilitators. Although the greatest proportion of time by far in experiential work is devoted to learners' discussion and exploration of their own communication skills, generalizing away from the interview in question, when handled sensitively, can help to make communication learning come alive. In Chapter 7 we describe how to achieve this in practice during experiential learning sessions. In addition, facilitators can link learners directly into the literature through reading assignments and project work.

ENDING

It is important that the feedback and analysis ends on a practical and constructive note. Time must be left to summarize the learning that has occurred, reiterate the skills that have been discussed and structure learning into a conceptual framework. As we have discussed, the use of the *Calgary–Cambridge observation guide* as a summarizing tool can be very helpful here. Rounds asking participants to summarize what they have learned and what next steps they intend to take are also of considerable value.

Using agenda-led, outcome-based analysis in other contexts

Agenda-led, outcome-based analysis is equally suited to work with real or simulated patients and with live or pre-recorded consultations. The method can also be used to explore role play between participants. Although we have described it here in the setting of small-group learning and primarily with the availability of video review, it can easily be adapted to the context of one-to one teaching and settings where video review is not available. In both these situations there are difficulties that need to be overcome; these, however, are not unique to agenda-led, outcome-based analysis but are common to all methods of providing feedback on the medical interview.

ONE-TO-ONE TEACHING

One-to-one teaching offers more time to individual learners. However, working in supportive peer groups with a skilled facilitator has two considerable advantages over one-to-one teaching: firstly it allows a far greater exchange of different approaches and secondly it enables easier rehearsal through role play.

In one-to-one teaching, only the learner and the facilitator are available to make offers and suggestions. As the number of different alternatives diminishes, it is easy to fall into the trap of simple disagreement and for a more defensive environment to be created between learner and teacher. Differences in power and knowledge complicate matters further. This is particularly true with the reluctant or less able learner who makes few suggestions. The facilitator finds himself speaking and offering suggestions to a passive non-contributor and the advantages of experiential learning rapidly diminish.

The advantages of receiving feedback from one's peers are lost. Whereas in small groups the facilitator makes suggestions or demonstrates a role play only after all the group members have contributed and only then if they have not solved the problem themselves, in one-to-one teaching the facilitator *is* the rest of the group and is forced to take a key role in the feedback process – the only two parties who can offer suggestions or demonstrate alternatives are the learner and the facilitator. At the same time, the facilitator must ensure a balance, manage defensiveness, support the learner, ask questions, deepen discussion and introduce cognitive material. The demands of being a key player in the feedback process make these other roles much more difficult to achieve.

Rehearsal is also more problematical in the one-to-one situation unless a simulated patient is available during feedback. Rather than having a dedicated group member to watch the interview from the patient's perspective and to role play the patient in subsequent rehearsal, learner and facilitator have to take turns to play the patient while the other tries out new ideas. This can work well but requires both facilitator and learner to be flexible – again a reluctant learner can easily sabotage the process and those in most need therefore lose out.

TEACHING WITHOUT VIDEO OR AUDIO REVIEW

Recordings enhance accurate and reliable self-assessment, a learner-centred approach, greater objectivity and more concrete, specific and descriptive feedback. Without recordings, it becomes even more important for observers to make detailed notes of the exact phrasing of comments and of observable behaviours so that an accurate record is available to support descriptive and specific feedback. The learner does not have the opportunity to replay the interview and observe his own performance. Therefore using the *Calgary–Cambridge observation guide* or anything else that helps structure observation and feedback, aid memory or increase the accuracy of feedback will be of value. Using agenda-led, outcome-based analysis in this situation requires little modification: we cannot use the recording to aid our discussions but instead must pay even more attention to the details of the rest of the method.

Phrasing feedback in communication skills teaching sessions

A key element of agenda-led, outcome-based analysis, as outlined above, is the use of descriptive feedback. We now continue our examination of 'how' to run an individual session by exploring descriptive feedback in depth. Agenda-led, outcome-based analysis provides an overall framework for structuring communication skills teaching while descriptive feedback specifies how to phrase feedback within that structure to ensure non-judgemental and specific comments.

Learners in medicine may rarely have experienced a learning situation involving observation where they have felt supported by a well-motivated teacher who is able to give non-judgemental yet constructive criticism (Ende *et al.* 1983; McKegney 1989; Westberg and Jason 1993). What guidelines can we advocate to both facilitators and group members to promote the phrasing of honest yet non-destructive feedback that the receiver can comfortably take on board?

Principles of constructive feedback

The following principles of constructive feedback are by no means new. They have been available for over a quarter of a century (Gibb 1961; Johnson 1972; Riccardi and Kurtz 1983; Silverman *et al.* 1997) yet have not infiltrated medical education to an appreciable extent. Even in communication skills teaching, an understanding of the principles of feedback is by no means universal.

FEEDBACK SHOULD BE DESCRIPTIVE RATHER THAN JUDGEMENTAL OR EVALUATIVE

Avoid phrasing feedback in terms of good or bad, right or wrong. Terms such as awful, stupid, brilliant, lazy and wonderful are of little value to the learner. Negative evaluation such as:

'The beginning was awful, you just seemed to ignore her'

is bound to create defensiveness. A judgement has been made that implies that the observer is comparing the person performing the interview to a set agreed standard against which the person has failed. Compare this with:

'At the beginning of the interview I noticed that you were facing the opposite direction looking at your notes which prevented eye contact between you.'

This is descriptive, non-judgemental feedback linked to outcome which is much easier to assimilate as a learner. It still points out the problem but in a way that is not seen as some deficiency of the learner. Similarly, positive evaluation is also unhelpful when provided judgementally:

'The beginning was excellent, great stuff.'

This does little to say why something was good and again implies a standard that has already been agreed upon. Contrast with:

'At the beginning, you gave her your full attention and never lost eye contact – your facial expression registered your interest in what she was saying.'

Communication skills are neither intrinsically good nor bad, they are simply helpful or not helpful in achieving a particular objective in a given situation. Because descriptive feedback is such a key component of constructive criticism, we elaborate on it in greater detail later in this chapter.

MAKE FEEDBACK SPECIFIC RATHER THAN GENERAL

General or vague comments such as:

'You didn't seem to be very empathic'

are not very helpful. Feedback should be detailed and specific. Focus on concrete descriptions of specific behaviour you can see and hear. Vague generalizations do not allow an entry point to looking at possible changes that might help the situation and may well only produce the reply *'Oh yes I was!'*. Contrast:

'Looking from the outside, I couldn't tell what you felt when she told you about her unhappiness. Your facial expression didn't change from when you were concentrating on her story – I felt she might not have known if you had heard or empathized with her.'

This leads constructively into looking at both the overall concept of empathy and the specific skills that allow patients to appreciate empathy overtly.

Use first person singular in giving feedback: 'I think …' rather than 'we think …' or 'most people think …'. Focus on your personal viewpoint and this particular situation rather than situations in general.

FOCUS FEEDBACK ON BEHAVIOUR RATHER THAN PERSONALITY

Describing someone as a *'loudmouth'* is a comment on an individual's personality – what you think he *is*. Saying *'You seemed to talk quite a lot, the patient tried to interrupt but couldn't quite get into the conversation'* is a comment on behaviour – what you think he *did*. Behaviour is easy to alter, personality less so; we are more likely to think we can change what we 'do' than what we 'are'.

FEEDBACK SHOULD BE FOR THE LEARNER'S BENEFIT

Patronizing, mocking, superior comments tend to benefit the observer rather than help and encourage the learner. Feedback should be given that serves the needs of the learner rather than the needs of the giver. It should not be simply a method of providing 'release' for the giver. Giving feedback that makes us feel better or gives us a psychological advantage serves only to be destructive to the learner and ultimately to the group as a whole.

FOCUS FEEDBACK ON SHARING INFORMATION RATHER THAN GIVING ADVICE

By sharing information we leave recipients of feedback free to decide for themselves what is the most appropriate course of action. In contrast, when we give advice we often tell others what to do and take away their freedom to decide for themselves; inadvertently we put them down. There is clearly a fine line in working with learners between sharing and giving advice, but we should move away from advice giving as a primary form of giving feedback towards the concept of generating alternatives, making offers and suggestions.

CHECK OUT INTERPRETATIONS OF FEEDBACK

Givers of feedback should take responsibility for checking out the consequences of their feedback. Just as in the consultation, be very conscious of the recipient's verbal and non-verbal reactions and overtly check out the response. We should be highly aware of the consequences of our feedback. In turn, the recipient should check out whether he has understood the feedback correctly: *'What I think you mean is ...'.* This prevents distortion and misunderstanding, which so easily occur if there is even a hint of defensiveness. Lastly, it is helpful for both giver and recipient to check out with the rest of the group to see if their impressions are shared by others.

LIMIT FEEDBACK TO THE AMOUNT OF INFORMATION THAT THE RECIPIENT CAN USE RATHER THAN THE AMOUNT WE WOULD LIKE TO GIVE

Overloading a person with feedback reduces the possibility that he will use any of it effectively. Again we may be satisfying some need of our own rather than helping the learner. We may feel that we have failed if we do not cover everything that we have seen rather than just concentrating for now on the most relevant areas for the learner. We must learn to trust that other opportunities to return to missed areas will arise later in the course – what is the point of covering everything now if it is not taken in by the learner?

FEEDBACK SHOULD BE SOLICITED RATHER THAN IMPOSED

Feedback is most usefully heard when the recipient has actively sought it and has asked for help with specific questions. We have already covered the importance of this concept in our discussion of agenda-led analysis. It is important for the group to have agreed in advance how and when feedback is to be given and received.

GIVE FEEDBACK ONLY ABOUT SOMETHING THAT CAN BE CHANGED

There is little point in reminding someone of a shortcoming that they cannot easily remedy. A nervous mannerism or a stutter may be a problem that can be acknowledged sensitively but detailed feedback about the mannerism itself may be unhelpful:

'If you didn't stutter so much, the patient would be able to understand you so much better. It's painfully slow for the patient.'

More useful would be:

'Obviously, the stutter is a problem you've had to live with over the years. Is there anything you'd like help with from the group with that or is it something you'd like us to accept and work around?'

Similarly, an organizational problem such as constant phone interruptions might be more difficult to change if the learner is a resident or student rather than the doctor in charge of the unit. Working on how to deal with interruptions rather than how to prevent them might be of more value to learners in these situations.

Descriptive feedback

How do we encourage learners to give appropriate feedback that conforms to the principles outlined above and that will positively enhance learning? The answer is descriptive feedback, a simple and easily understood approach which naturally allows feedback to be:

- non-judgemental
- specific
- directed towards behaviour rather than personality
- well intentioned
- sharing
- checked with the recipient.

Descriptive feedback is the process of holding a mirror up for the group. Instead of *'what was done well'* and *'what could have been done differently'*, we substitute

- *'Here's what I saw or heard'*
- *'What do you think?'*

By describing exactly what you saw in the interview, you almost always produce non-evaluative specific feedback. An example is required here to demonstrate the power of the method: if a patient starts to look down, fiddles with her fingers, slows down her speech and looks weepy, and the interviewer then asks her how her family is getting on to which she responds that she is fine, regains her equanimity and never returns to why she looked so uncomfortable, you could give feedback in two different ways:

'I think you really missed a big cue when she obviously had something important to say and you chickened out of asking her.'

This is judgemental, general feedback that assumes a motive for the learner's actions with an implied comment on his personality.

'At 3 minutes 23 seconds, there was an interesting point when she starts to look down, fiddles with her fingers, slows down her speech and looks weepy. You then asked her about her family and she didn't ever seem to get back to what was upsetting her. What do you think, John?'

'Yes, I didn't know quite how to get her to open up.'

This is descriptive feedback that is non-judgemental and very specific. It also very effectively leads the discussion on into what outcome you are trying to achieve. If the learner in question in fact did not wish to enter the realm of the patient's feelings because he was an hour behind, then what he did achieved his ends. He can own the thoughts and feelings that were contributing to his actions. However, even so the group could practise at this point how they might get the patient to open up if they had enough time on another occasion or they could consider alternatives that take the patient's point of view into account.

Notice how descriptive feedback concentrates initially on *what*, *when*, *where* and *how* rather than *why*. Comments on 'why' something was done move from the observable to the inferred and can easily lead into the more contentious territory of assumptions about motives and actions (Premi 1991).

Here are two examples: note that *positive* feedback also benefits from description that is concrete and specific. Compare:

'I think you were great the way you got the patient to tell his story so easily' (general and not very helpful in learning)

with

'You asked her when it started and then let her talk. Whenever she seemed to stop, you waited a few seconds and said "uh huh" and she continued her tale. She told you all about her problem and her fears in her own words'

or:

'That was awful, you just lectured her'

with

'When you explained the condition to her, you gave her a lot of information and talked in some detail for two minutes without pause. She didn't ask any questions but I noticed that she frowned after about 40 seconds. What do you think, John?'

Note how well descriptive feedback fits in with the principles of agenda-led, outcome-based analysis. Firstly, reflection back to the learner being observed allows self-problem solving. Secondly, description of what happened leads on directly to what effect it seemed to have; this in turn leads on to what the learner or group wish had happened and what outcome they would like to have achieved. Finally, the group can consider what skills would be helpful in enabling them to get there.

The aim of descriptive feedback is to:

- reduce defensiveness
- promote open discussion
- increase experimentation
- aid the presentation and consideration of available alternatives
- ultimately facilitate change in behaviour.

By trying to be more descriptive, we are attempting to create a non-judgemental climate that encourages learning. Of course, some judgement is involved in the very act of selecting what area to describe; there is a selective perceptual bias in all that we do. But by moving our language away from the judgemental framework of good and bad and into the descriptive framework of *'what we saw'*, we change the way feedback is received and possibly even the way that we think. If the observer has formed a judgement, she should hold back from the use of evaluative language so that the receiver of feedback can make use of the descriptive information himself without becoming defensive. This is not to say that analysis and interpretation should never feature but that the person doing the interview should be given every chance to make inferences himself first. If this is not fruitful then it may be appropriate to move into a slightly more interpretive mode. Here is an example of this graded approach.

Jane: *'You asked four questions in quick succession and the patient just answered yes or no.'*
Facilitator: *'What do you think, John?'*

Now if John answers *'I think that I got some useful information with those questions'* rather than *'Yes, I felt it was very hard going'*, you could proceed as follows:

Facilitator: *'Can I just return to what you were saying Jane. What were you thinking about John's questions, what effect did you think they had?'*
Jane: *'I think John's closed questions led the patient just to give answers rather than tell his story.'*

Note that in the above example, Jane has still used non-judgemental language without reference to good or bad but has moved slightly along the path of analysis by inferring cause and effect.

The 'SET–GO' method of descriptive, outcome-based feedback

Box 5.3   The 'SET–GO' method of descriptive feedback

Group members to base their feedback on:

1 *'What I **S**aw'*
   (descriptive, specific, non-judgemental)

Facilitator prompts if necessary with either or both of:

2 *'What **E**lse did you see?'*
   (what happened next in descriptive terms)
3 *'What do you **T**hink, John?'*
   (reflecting back to the person doing the interview who is then given an opportunity to acknowledge and problem solve himself)

Facilitator then gets the whole group to problem solve:

1 *'Can we clarify what **G**oal we would like to achieve?'*
   (outcome-based approach)

2 *'Any **O**ffers of how we should get there?'*
   (suggestions, alternatives to be rehearsed if possible)

Descriptive feedback therefore enables and encourages non-judgemental, specific feedback directed towards behaviour rather than personality and linked to thoughts and feelings. How can the facilitator encourage this process to occur within agenda-led, outcome-based analysis? To help facilitators combine the principles of descriptive feedback and an outcome-based approach, we have developed an easily remembered guide that can be handed to participants, encapsulated by the mnemonic 'SET-GO' (Silverman *et al.* 1997) (Box 5.3).

The facilitator's task then becomes one of raising awareness of the outcome-based approach.

- *'When you asked how her family were getting on, can I clarify what were you aiming for, what you were trying to achieve?'*
- *'Can you think of any alternatives that might have helped her to voice what was upsetting her?'*
- *'Let's work on that a little – can anyone else think of a way in here?'*

This allows the facilitator to get the group to go back one stage, focus more on outcomes and be more open to alternatives. It also allows the facilitator to counter participants' inappropriately judgemental feedback with ease by linking the feedback to description or outcome. If a group member says *'That was awful'*, instead of saying *'Hold on a minute, you can't say that'*, you can ask *'When you say awful, could you describe exactly what didn't work for you? What did you see?'* or *'Can you say what you would have liked to achieve and then we can work out how to get there?'*

6

Running a session: facilitation tools to maximize participation and learning

Introduction

Chapter 5 described an approach to facilitation that provides a secure platform for learning and improving communication skills. This chapter focuses on additional facilitation tools which help to create a supportive climate for learning and maximize participation. These are essential elements of any learning leading to skill development and personal change and are therefore of particular importance in experiential communication skills programmes.

We also address how to deal with difficult situations. In spite of our best efforts, sooner or later all of us who facilitate or participate in communication programmes are bound to face uncomfortable challenges or come up against barriers to learning that we are not sure how to handle such as defensiveness, cynicism, lack of confidence, disagreements, mistakes or poor performance. Here, we present a variety of skills and strategies for meeting such challenges.

In this chapter we:

- relate effective facilitation to effective communication with patients and show how the same skills and principles form a common foundation for both
- offer a series of concepts, models and strategies that are helpful in developing a supportive environment and maximizing participation and learning
- present strategies for dealing with difficult situations and tensions to advantage.

Facilitation and learning are enhanced if both facilitators *and* learners understand and use the tools and resources outlined in this chapter, since communication training with its heavy reliance on peer teaching and self-assessment makes 'teachers' of us all. Mastering this material pays double dividends – it is just as applicable to interactions with patients and colleagues in professional practice as it is to interactions with learners.

Relating facilitation to communication with patients

The parallel between communication skills and facilitation skills

Effective communication is at the root of effective facilitation. In fact, the skills required to communicate effectively with patients are so similar to those required for teaching that the *Calgary–Cambridge observation guide* serves equally well as a summary of both communication and facilitation skills. To transform the guide into a concise skills manual and self-assessment tool for facilitators, simply substitute 'facilitator' and 'learner' for 'physician' and 'patient' throughout.

Physicians exploring the skills of facilitation are often relieved to discover that they are building on a familiar base of skills and structures which they already use when talking with patients:

- **getting the session started** (as we discuss later in this chapter) – *parallel to initiating the consultation*
- **structuring the group's learning** – discovering learners' agendas and the outcomes they want to reach (as discussed in 'Agenda-led, outcome-based analysis' in Chapter 5); using summary, signposting – *parallel to structuring the consultation during initiation and information gathering*
- **facilitation through questions and responses** – open questions, attentive listening, encouragement, silence, repetition, paraphrasing, interpretation, clarification, internal summary, sharing of thoughts, discovering the learners' ideas, beliefs and expectations (as discussed in 'Motivating participation, thinking and learning' later in this chapter) – *parallel to gathering information in the consultation*
- **building the relationship** – acceptance, empathy, support, sensitivity, picking up cues (part of supportive climate and among the key elements for dealing with defended and conflicted situations skills, as discussed later in this chapter) – *parallel to building the relationship in the consultation*
- **providing information** (as discussed in Chapter 7) – *parallel to explanation and planning in the consultation.*

The parallel between the principles of effective communication and the principles of effective facilitation

In Chapter 2 we identified five principles that characterize effective communication. These principles apply equally well to effective facilitation and provide a framework to help us decide how best to facilitate learning in the communication skills curriculum. Thinking now in terms of facilitating learning rather than communicating with patients, we can ask ourselves what we did in any given session to:

- ensure interaction (between learners and facilitator, among learners)
- reduce uncertainty appropriately (about what to expect, the session's agenda, whether the group or we can be trusted)

- demonstrate dynamism (involvement, flexibility and responsiveness)
- help learners to think in terms of outcomes and consequences (what are you aiming for, what happened)
- apply the helical model (build in repetition and review, encourage learners to take their 'next steps' in the spiral process of mastering skills and understanding).

We introduce these principles to learners as a framework for effective group participation. For example, the helix becomes a useful model for how to learn skills. Most of us progress up the learning spiral for a time and then fall back down temporarily, perhaps when we try to apply an 'old' skill in a new context or suffer a setback in our confidence. The group benefits from understanding that such apparent setbacks, though uncomfortable, are often the prelude to significant leaps forward.

Westberg and Jason (1993) offer another set of principles which characterize helpful teacher–learner relationships. Again, note the crossover with effective doctor–patient communication:

- openness and honesty
- mutual trust
- mutual respect
- support and nurture
- collaboration, fostering the learner's independence
- flexibility
- constant evolution.

It takes time to create trusting relationships and to build credibility as a facilitator. Like patients, many learners are used to adopting passive roles with their teachers and find it difficult to abandon familiar patterns and move to a more collaborative model. This is also true of facilitators who may be more familiar with an authoritarian approach. Most doctors have had to be competitive in their careers and have witnessed the competition which dominates relationships in the medical profession at all levels. It is not surprising if the shift to collaboration and cooperation is difficult at first. But if facilitators apply the skills and principles described throughout this chapter and encourage learners to do the same, the effect will be increased collaboration, enhanced learning and the prevention of many potential difficulties both within the group and between facilitators and learners.

Strategies for maximizing participation and learning

Optimal learning and skill development occur in a climate of trust and openness as opposed to mistrust and defensiveness. Unfortunately, when learning requires us to reassess or even challenge our beliefs and ideas, to learn new skills or to change the way we do things, some degree of defensiveness and conflict is inevitable. Tension produced by the realization that there is a need for change often acts as a potent motivating force for learning: it shakes us out of our comfortable complacency. However, this very discomfort can just as easily be channelled into defensiveness. Learners can react by blocking and digging in their heels, spending their attention and energy on protecting themselves or reducing perceived threats instead of on learning and change.

Given this reality, creating a supportive environment is essential for any communication skills course. But support, like challenge, is not enough. Support without challenge can be comfortable but invites collusion and limits progress; challenge without support is potentially destructive. So what can we do to develop and maintain a supportive learning climate? How do we get the balance right between enabling learners to experience the *frisson* of discomfort required to edge them forward in their learning and simultaneously providing them with the support necessary to flourish? And how do we deal with defensiveness and potential conflict when they do inevitably arise?

Building a supportive climate

In this section we explore two closely related strategies for developing and maintaining a supportive climate and maximizing participation in experiential learning. We then provide a set of practical guidelines for establishing a supportive environment at the beginning of each course and session.

GIBB'S STRATEGIES FOR SUPPORTIVE VERSUS DEFENSIVE CLIMATE

Helping to create safety and a supportive climate are important tasks for everyone in the group but the facilitator has particular responsibility for leadership in this area and for dealing with any difficulties that crop up despite everyone's best efforts. The work of Gibb (1961) is a particularly useful resource for creating and then maintaining a supportive climate, for reducing defensiveness to manageable levels when it does appear and for restoring a supportive climate and safety when they are temporarily compromised. Based on an eight-year study which looked at audiotaped recordings of small-group discussions, Gibb identified six categories of behaviour that are characteristic of a supportive climate in groups (first item in each pair below) and six alternative categories that are characteristic of a defensive climate (second item in each pair). It is not difficult to guess which set of categories describes the stereotype of the traditional authoritarian teacher.

Supportive climate	*Defensive climate*
1 **Description** Non-judgemental presentation of perceptions, feelings, events; genuine requests for information; descriptively reflecting opinions and direct observations of visible behaviour back to the other person; avoiding terms like 'good' or 'bad'	**Evaluation** Passing judgement; blaming, criticizing *or* praising; questioning motives or standards
2 **Problem orientation** Collaboration; mutually defining and solving problems rather than telling someone what to do	**Control** Doing something to other people; telling them what to do or how to feel or think
3 **Spontaneity** (flexibility) Freedom from 'hidden agendas' or other deceptions; straightforwardness; the ability to respond to events and people with	**Strategy** (hidden agenda) Manipulating through the use of tricks or hidden plans; hiding intentions

flexibility. Spontaneity should not be construed to mean lack of organization or absence of plans and structure

4 **Empathy** (involvement)
Willingness to become involved with others; identifying with, respecting, accepting, understanding others

Neutrality (indifference)
Indifference, detachment, aloofness; viewing the other person as an object of study

5 **Equality**
Willingness to participate with the other person, to mutually define and solve problems; de-emphasis of differences in power or ability. Equality does not deny differences in knowledge or ability, rather it recognizes the contribution and worth of each individual

Superiority
Failure to recognize the worth of the other person, arousing feelings of inadequacy in the other; communicating that one is better than the other

6 **Provisionalism** (tentativeness)
Tentativeness; open-mindedness; willingness to explore alternative points of view or plans of action

Certainty (dogmatism)
Dogmatism; resisting consideration of alternatives; emphasis on proving a point rather than solving the problem

To develop and maintain a supportive climate – and thereby open the way for learning or change – consciously employ description, problem orientation, spontaneity, empathy, equality and provisionalism and avoid as much as possible evaluation, control, strategy, neutrality, superiority and certainty (as defined by Gibb). This is the framework we turn to first whenever we are starting with a group and when difficulties of any kind arise that we are not sure how to handle. We find this framework particularly useful as a means for coping with defensiveness and distrust whenever these attitudes appear in learning or health care settings.

Creating a supportive climate is, however, more complex than simply using supportive and avoiding defensive climate behaviours. Although the definitions of the defensive categories focus on their negative side, these categories are not always inappropriate. Evaluation and control are appropriate under some circumstances regardless of the defensiveness that may result. The level of defensiveness already present will influence the degree to which the various categories will generate defensiveness or supportiveness. If the group has developed a supportive climate then participants are freer to make and more easily tolerate comments in any of the categories. On the other hand, if defensiveness begins to block learning, intentionally go back to using the supportive categories. And certainly these are the preferred starting points in all unknown or new situations.

MUTUALLY UNDERSTOOD COMMON GROUND: THE BASIS FOR TRUST AND RELATIONSHIPS

A model derived from Baker's (1955) work gives us another tool for creating a supportive climate, encouraging participation and dealing with defensiveness. The model underscores the significance of what Baker calls 'reciprocal identification' or, as we have labelled it, 'mutually understood common ground' (Riccardi and Kurtz 1983). According to Baker, the effectiveness

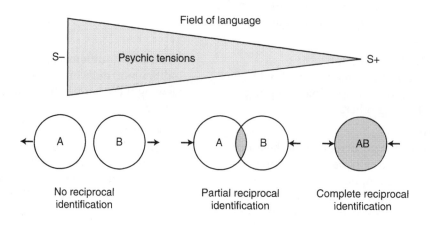

Fig 6.1 Baker (1955) model of communication.

of any communication (or teaching effort) is dependent on the degrees of commonality between the communicators, the extent to which one person in an interaction can accurately identify with the other. More recent work corroborates this hypothesis. For example, in a study of 315 patients and their 39 primary care physicians, Stewart *et al.* (1997) found the 'patient's perception of finding common ground with the physician' to be associated with better patient recovery from their discomfort and concern, better emotional health two months after being seen and fewer lab tests and referrals. Roter's (1997) work on the merit of mutuality and partnership also reinforces the concept that 'common ground' is significant to physician–patient communication just as it is to small-group teaching and learning. A closer look at Baker's model (Fig. 6.1) provides insight about why this is so.

Circles A and B in Fig. 6.1 represent two people interacting, while the shaded overlapping area represents the degree of mutually understood common ground between them. Some mutually understood commonality exists, for example, if both A and B share a common culture or language *and* if *both* know that to be the case. Identification of common ground on the part of only one individual is not enough. The commonalities must be *reciprocally* identified, that is, *mutually* understood. Additional mutually understood common ground may be developed as A and B reveal their backgrounds, goals, beliefs, etc. to each other through communication (i.e. 'field of language') and as they share time and experiences together. Such reciprocal identification is a significant basis for trust and accuracy.

How participants feel during pauses or periods of silence is an indicator of their reciprocal identification. In the model, S– represents uncomfortable silence which is accompanied by higher levels of tension and corresponds to a relative lack of mutually understood common ground (e.g. due to conflict, embarrassment, defensiveness); S+ represents comfortable silence which is accompanied by lower tension and reflects higher degrees of reciprocal identification (e.g. due to shared understanding and lack of defensiveness). The model assists us in determining the degree of rapport or mutually understood common ground existing in a relationship at any given moment.

The last phrase 'at any given moment' is important. The degree of reciprocal identification is in constant flux. While achievement, even momentarily, of complete reciprocal identification can have a continuing positive effect on a relationship, there is no guarantee that the relationship will continue in that state. A new misunderstanding or conflict can temporarily throw any relationship (or group) back to negative silence and a perception of no reciprocal identification. The solution suggested by this model is to re-establish a degree of trust by returning to a point where common ground can again be mutually recognized (for example, both parties agree that they want to stay in the relationship) and then work to redevelop mutually understood common ground from there (for example, about a description of the problem that both can agree on).

How does Baker's model help us?

- It emphasizes that one way to reduce tension, deal with misunderstanding and create a supportive climate is to establish common points of reference, for example through developing jointly agreed upon objectives.
- It gives us a useful method for establishing trust, building relationships and encouraging participation – doing anything that helps establish mutually understood common ground.
- It offers a partial explanation for the discomfort many of us experience during even short silences in an unfamiliar group or with an individual with whom we have little rapport or some sort of current misunderstanding.
- It offers a way to reduce such discomfort, namely by sharing experience or attempting to (re)establish common ground.

As we facilitate, reflect and offer feedback, we find it useful to keep two more ideas in mind that are related to common ground. First, *effective communication (or teaching) is not the same as telling nor does hearing mean that we have understood*. Accurate communication cannot be assumed just because a message has been sent or heard. We cannot rely on what for most purposes is false logic: I assume that I see X accurately; I assume that you see X accurately; therefore, I assume that you see X the same way that I see X (or vice versa) (Schutz 1967). Feedback and discussion that lead to *mutually* understood common ground are essential to effective communication.

Second, *communication is not the same as agreement*. Many of us erroneously assume that our communication – or our facilitation – has 'broken down' or been misunderstood if others end up disagreeing with our point of view. But disagreement is not the same as misunderstanding. In fact, disagreement may well be the result of exemplary communication. The mutually understood common ground that we achieve may be simply an accurate understanding of each other's quite different points of view and an agreement to accept the differences as valid and acceptable. This perspective is useful when people disagree about the 'best' way to proceed – often you can diffuse the disagreement and save considerable time by pointing out that consensus is not necessary, that it is helpful to hear alternative points of view. Energy is better spent on accurately understanding alternatives than on arguing over which alternative is best.

GETTING STARTED: LAYING THE FOUNDATIONS FOR A SUPPORTIVE ENVIRONMENT

An important opportunity to lay the foundations for a supportive environment occurs at the very first meeting with new learners and again at the beginning of each session. Many of the suggestions that we propose for getting started are practical ways to ensure that we put into practice Gibb's (1961) supportive climate behaviours and Baker's (1955) model of establishing mutually understood common ground. Here again, there is a parallel between the learning session and the consultation. Consider the striking resemblance between the skills of initiating the session in the *Calgary–Cambridge observation guide* and those in the following list which pertain to getting started with learners:

- preparation
- establishing initial rapport
  - demonstrating interest and respect, modelling appropriate behaviours
  - introductions: self and participants
  - getting acquainted, building trust
  - settling in, leaving preoccupations behind
- developing a culture of safety and support
  - explicit contracting of ground rules
  - discussing intentions and responsibilities
- sharing and negotiating agendas
  - setting clear prior objectives (no secret agendas)
  - discovering the learners' needs and agendas
  - negotiating the agenda, taking both learners' and facilitators' needs and ideas into account.

Preparation. The key to facilitator confidence and comfort is good preparation. Prepare materials, equipment and the meeting place before learners arrive.

Establishing initial rapport. If we wish learners to behave with trust, respect, openness, honesty, empathy, gentleness, humour, sensitivity and friendliness, we need to model these qualities and demonstrate interest and respect ourselves.

Introductions, including backgrounds and name preferences, are a good place to start if the learning group is not acquainted. Introductions can include brief warm-up or ice-breaking exercises to enable participants to get to know each other by sharing their backgrounds or experience. Even when we join groups briefly that have been meeting for some time, for example to substitute for an absent facilitator, we begin with a few minutes where we invite everyone to give us an idea of who they are, for instance, by saying something about themselves that others are not likely to know already. This opportunity to listen, respond, laugh together and whenever possible to connect by establishing mutually understood common ground (regarding hometowns, family, similar pastimes, etc.) sets the foundation for trust and supportive climate with remarkable ease. Exercises can also be used to enable participants to settle in and leave their preoccupations behind. As with all getting started activities, we consider ourselves a bona fide group member who contributes like any other member.

Developing a culture of safety and support. The next step is to ask learners what ground rules they want to put in place for how the group will run. These may relate to ensuring everyone's right to speak and be heard, establishing rules of confidentiality, promoting honest and constructive rather than destructive criticism, calling time out during a consultation to get assistance, attendance policies, etc. This, like introductions, begins to develop norms for collaboration, shared decision making and openness within the group.

Discussing intentions and responsibilities may seem obvious but often these are not made overt. Try being explicit with what you are prepared to offer to your learners at the beginning of a course or session. For example, say that you wish to model equality, remain a learner, facilitate humour and try to pick up and acknowledge all they say; that you intend to offer choices and alternatives, admit fallibility, etc. Ask learners to correct you if you get it wrong. Emphasize that maintaining a supportive climate, like learning, is ultimately a responsibility shared by everyone in the group. Talk about the benefits of every group member learning about how to facilitate each other's learning; encourage them to read Chapters 5 and 6 of this book.

Sharing and negotiating agendas. Setting clear prior objectives for the session or course is helpful as it reduces unnecessary uncertainty. How you advertise a course or session is important; it can help learners know exactly what to expect. Clearly structured course objectives can be distributed before the course begins along with information of who will be facilitating, the rationale for the course, its length and methods that will be used.

When we meet learners we ask them to identify the goals and objectives that they wish to work on, to establish their learning needs and agendas. With learners who are meeting for the first or second time, we focus on long-term goals. For example, we give learners a brief time to jot down their personal goals and then share them with the group, perhaps working first in pairs or trios. Hearing each other's ideas usually leads to changes and additions in personal goals and the emergence of common ground regarding shared goals. These lists are flexible; as the course proceeds learners will undoubtedly alter their original thinking. Later on in the course we may bring out a collation of these original lists to encourage learners to continue thinking in terms of the outcomes they wish to attain.

Usually at the end of the discussion of goals, we review the objectives which course organizers have 'set' for the course, comparing to see where there is overlap and where the group's individual or shared goals differ. This discussion may well result in changes to the preplanned course goals. Just as with patients, we then negotiate a shared agenda for the course.

After discussing long-term goals, shift to short-term goals held in common for a given session (e.g. those set at a previous meeting or preplanned by course organizers) as well as those which an individual learner has for her specific consultation – we may ask for the latter both before the consultation ('Anything in particular you want us to watch for?') and after ('Anything in particular you'd like us to focus on during the discussion?').

We then discuss how the group wishes to proceed, given the outcomes they wish to achieve. If we are new to an already formed group, we ask how they usually do things so that we can follow that pattern or ask if the group would be willing to try an alternative approach.

During the first session these activities will take some time. Thereafter, we generally need take only a few minutes at the start of each session to re-establish a supportive environment and identify goals. This effort is, however, crucial to the success of the session as a whole.

Motivating participation, thinking and learning throughout the session

Once the session has started well and the foundations of a supportive climate and collaborative learning are in place, two important facilitation tools are necessary to maximize learners' involvement and participation: responding techniques and questioning techniques. Just as with patients in the consultation, the way you respond to learners' comments, the way you invite them to participate and the questions you ask are key factors in determining the outcome of a session. These techniques correspond directly to the information-gathering skills of the consultation listed in the *Calgary–Cambridge observation guide* and elaborated upon in our companion title, *Skills for Communicating with Patients*.

RESPONDING

The skills of listening and responding to learners are central to effective facilitation. They are identical to the following skills used in the consultation:

- attentive listening
- encouragement
- silence
- repetition
- paraphrasing
- interpretation
- clarification
- internal summary
- picking up verbal and non-verbal cues.

These responding skills are also the key skills of non-directive counselling. They have been extensively discussed by Rogers (1980), Egan (1990) and others and are accepted as crucial elements of any communication which aims to encourage the client to talk more about their problem without undue professional direction.

For examples of responding techniques that work we turn to a qualitative study (Kurtz 1990) involving several days' observation of one doctor during his bedside-attending rounds. Learners perceived him to be particularly effective in his ability to stimulate participation, lateral thinking and learning. Not surprisingly, the study revealed that question and response techniques were among his key skills. Here, we look at the listening and responding skills that he used to stimulate participation and learning. At every opportunity he employed techniques that acknowledged and reinforced learners:

- choosing silence as a response, accompanied by obvious concentration; focusing intently on whoever is speaking
- repeating or reiterating learner comments thoughtfully: *'So you'd be thinking about…'*; *'So she gets to go home for Christmas with her kids'*
- picking up verbal and non-verbal cues: *'You're looking tired today … let's break after this'*
- interrupting infrequently: when necessary, giving non-verbal cues first such as moving forward slightly and establishing eye contact
- reinforcing learners' ideas, reacting out loud: *'That's a good suggestion'*; *'Hmm … Oh …'*; *'Your instincts are right.'*; *'OK. I understand a lot better now'*
- waiting three to five seconds after a question to give learners time to think and respond
- asking for specific clarification: *'Could you explain what you mean by …'*
- paraphrasing to check interpretation: *'So what you are most concerned about is whether …'*

QUESTIONING

Three basic types of questions are useful in facilitation:

1 **open**, for which many responses are possible

2 **closed**, which require only a word or two as a response and which usually have only one right answer
3 **Socratic**, which follow Socrates' pattern of asking small questions that open the way for learners to 'discover' answers themselves.

All are appropriate at various times, depending on the outcomes you wish to achieve. For engaging learners and encouraging participation and lateral thinking, open and Socratic questions are the most effective.

We return to the above study of one doctor during his attending rounds. Here, we look at his questioning techniques. In general, he used questions to challenge his small group of medical students and residents to think further or integrate information differently. Using variations of Socratic questioning most frequently, he gave the impression of 'thinking with' rather than testing or evaluating learners, of jointly working to solve problems or come up with alternatives. The following specific examples from his facilitation demonstrate how to question more effectively:

- asking questions in the context of what learners are doing; reiteration, then: *'So what are you thinking about at this point?'*
- explicitly inviting learners' questions throughout: *'Any more questions?'*; *'Anything else we need to know ...?'*
- pushing learners to think beyond their initial responses, sometimes giving them an idea of the next appropriate step: *'What else do you want to know?'*; *'What would you do to find out if that would work?'*
- using questions to give learners the opportunity to teach what they know to each other: *'Did you see a recent study reported in ...? Want to tell us about it?'*
- inviting learners out loud to think along with you, especially after asking them a series of related questions to get at something you are puzzling about or that they had overlooked. After a few questions, step back and ask: *'What am I working on?'*
- implying questions and/or getting thinking started by offering an opinion: *'Here's what I think ... What do you think?'*
- using questions to raise alternative perspectives, to show learners how the assumptions they make can lead them astray: *'So you're assuming the patient is manipulating the doctor. If you assume instead that what the patient's doing is a reasonable reaction to the problem (or reasonable considering the narcotic doses we're giving her), then what do you think?'*
- inviting learners to guess when no one has an answer: *'Would you like to guess?'*

The doctor used a further technique – thinking out loud – for both questioning and responding. He thereby made his thinking and problem solving visible to learners (and patients). Examples include:

- frequently revealing thinking with appropriately timed remarks like: *'Here's my problem. We have the disease nailed but we need to determine how we can help her function best with the time she has left.'* (Learners responded by admitting that they needed more information; they had focused on details of history and diagnosis and had missed the patient's perspective and the point of the care she needed now)
- summarizing frequently, interrupting with questions that occur to you as you summarize
- inviting learners to 'help you out', to answer the questions you are working on in your own mind: *'What I'm thinking is ... How are we going to resolve this problem?'*

Models of learning and change

This section describes several models of learning and change which demonstrate the stages learners pass through in developing new skills and patterns of behaviour. An appreciation of these models contributes to the development of a supportive climate by helping learners and facilitators become more realistic in their expectations and thus more comfortable and less defensive in learning situations.

FOUR-STAGE MODEL OF LEARNING

The four-stage model of learning (Wackman *et al.* 1976) describes four stages that individuals progress through when learning any new skill. Just telling learners about this model has a positive effect, perhaps because it gives them licence to admit to, and even joke about, the stages as they progress through them. Once learners understand that experiencing each stage is natural and expected, they gain a freedom to move in and out of the stages – to make mistakes, go forward, regress, recover – with minimal defensiveness and more grace.

The stages may make more sense if you apply them first to a physical or artistic skill that you have already mastered. Try to recall what it was like to learn to swim or play an instrument, especially if you learned as an adult.

1 *Beginning awareness stage.* Characterized by confusion and excitement, this stage involves a recognition that there are ways of doing things which you may never even have thought of, much less mastered. Motivation is not a significant problem as everything is still new and different.
2 *Awkward stage.* At this stage you have increased awareness of new skills or approaches but are experiencing difficulty using them. You feel clumsy, mechanical, phoney, awkward, as though you are just not being 'yourself'. You may complain about becoming too self-conscious and tend to blame your instructor or fellow learners for your apparent lack of progress. In this stage your behaviour may seem forced, spontaneity will be reduced and you feel generally ill at ease.
3 *Consciously skilful stage.* You are still quite self-conscious at this stage but are beginning to use the skills more effectively. You feel more comfortable and begin to adapt the new skills to your own personal style. Nevertheless, your actions remain somewhat mechanical and you still have to think carefully about what you are doing.
4 *Integrated stage.* It takes time, continued effort and practice to reach this stage. Here you will feel comfortable, competent and spontaneous as you use the new skills. They will have become a part of your natural behaviour.

In real life, this progression is not irreversible. Regression is likely, particularly when you are under stress, tired, distracted by unrelated personal problems or trying to apply newly de- veloped skills in contexts which are new to you. Fortunately, once you do reach the integrated stage you regress less frequently even when tensions increase or a new context presents itself.

An additional note about the awkward stage is warranted. When you first enter this stage or later regress to it, you may find yourself coming up with any number of excuses for not continuing to experiment with, much less adopt, new behaviours. Some of our favourites in the communication skills setting include:

- *'This is phoney, it just isn't "me".'*
- *'This all makes me too self-conscious.'*
- *'Communication training is a crock.'*
- *'Once you're an adult your communication patterns and ways of relating are formed and that's that.'*
- *'I can learn this stuff later, on my own, when nobody is around observing.'*
- *'I may not be great but I'm good enough.'*

We share the four-stage model with our participants early on and revisit it at opportune moments. For example, to allay avoidance or withdrawal tactics such as those above, we review the model and urge our participants to keep at it until they feel at ease with a 'new' behaviour, that is, at least until reaching the consciously skilled stage.

This model reduces defensiveness by making us more realistic in our expectations of ourselves and others and more patient about the time it takes for lasting behaviour changes to develop. The model also explains the necessity for repeated rehearsal, observation and feedback. Think of the tennis player who can play reasonably well but goes for a lesson with a professional to improve his skills. The professional observes, notices problems with the angle of the racquet on the forehand drive and suggests a change in grip. Now, instead of playing reasonably, every shot is a disaster, even ones the learner used to play well. He is thinking so hard about each shot that all his spontaneity is reduced and he feels worse than when he started. Only further rehearsal, feedback and encouragement will allow him to assimilate the new approach into the rest of his game so that he can improve. Eventually, his game will feel natural and improved. He will have reached the fourth stage.

REFRAMING OUR THINKING ABOUT OUTCOMES

It is easy to assume that teaching and learning are successful only if participants actually accomplish a change in their behaviour. In place of this somewhat limiting notion, it is helpful to consider the different outcomes or kinds of change that facilitators can aim for.

Outcomes of change. Rather than thinking only in terms of action, consider these four alternative outcomes:

- consideration (I am aware of and willing to consider change)
- attitudes (I have a positive attitude toward the change)
- beliefs and values (I believe the change is the best approach)
- action/behaviour (I change the way I act or behave in real life).

If we assess where in this progression learners are, we can understand more precisely where to direct our efforts and what 'next steps' to move toward. Of course, our ultimate aim is to achieve change in behaviour and improvement in learners' skills. But a more indirect approach often results in less defensiveness and proves more fruitful than trying to influence action immediately. If I am not yet even willing to consider a change, I am less likely to make a lasting change in behaviour than if I already have a positive attitude toward the change.

Thinking in terms of four outcomes instead of one (i.e. action) changes the way we assess our teaching efforts and learners' progress. It allows us to record advancement not only when we can see changes in behaviour but also when we can see changes in what learners are willing to consider, in their attitude or in what they believe and value.

The stages of change model. Compare this model with Prochaska and DiClementi's (1986) more recent stages of change model, which they apply to addictive behaviour:

– pre-contemplation
– contemplation
– active change
– maintenance
– relapse (and circling back through the earlier stages)
or
– success.

Recognizing these naturally occurring stages and helping clients or learners to understand which stage they have reached assists in determining how to support or influence motivation and progress.

Conviction and confidence. Keller and Kemp White (1997) identify two additional factors that significantly influence outcomes related to motivation and change:

• conviction
  – how important is this change to you?
  – how committed are you?
• confidence
  – how confident are you that you know how (have skills) to make this change?
  – how likely do you think it is that you will make this change?

Each factor simultaneously helps determine and create readiness to change. Keller and Kemp White express the interactive relationship between conviction and confidence in terms of a grid (Fig. 6.2) which provides a means for 'quantifying' levels of conviction and confidence

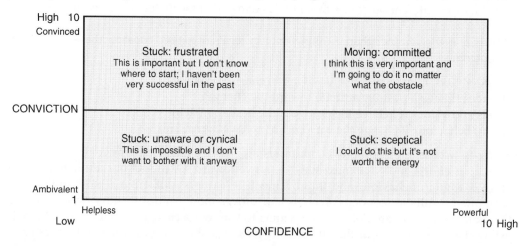

Fig 6.2 Conviction and confidence grid (Keller and Kemp White 1997).

and describes how people get stuck in their attempts to change. They apply their model in conjunction with Prochaska and DiClementi's (1986) stages of change model. In helping patients to make lifestyle changes or follow treatment regimens, clinicians need to find out not only which stage of change their clients are in with respect to each change or new behaviour but also where clients are on the conviction/confidence grid. Different positions on the grid call for clinicians to use different techniques in assisting their patients with change. Keller and Kemp White also encourage clinicians to use the grid as a means of assessing their own conviction and commitment to helping patients and their own motivation to change personal or professional behaviour.

The conviction/confidence grid pertains equally well to learning new communication (or facilitation) skills ourselves or to helping others to do so. This book and its companion volume focus on increasing not only readers' competence but also their conviction and confidence with respect to the 'why', 'what' and 'how' of communication skills teaching and learning. Our approach to facilitation and communication in medicine also intentionally aims to protect and enhance learners', patients' and doctors' self-esteem, a factor which underlies confidence and conviction.

Combining the conviction/confidence grid and considerations of self-esteem with the four-stage model of learning (beginning awareness, awkward, consciously skilled, integrated) and the outcomes of change model (consideration, attitudes, beliefs, action) deepens the usefulness of all three approaches. Seen in this light, heightened conviction, confidence and self-esteem are *outcomes* worth working on in communication programmes as well as means to an end.

Strategies for dealing with difficulties

Responding to defended and conflicted situations: the basics

There will always be occasions when the supportive environment you have carefully engendered breaks down. Here, we present a set of facilitation skills to use when learners either challenge each other or the facilitator, particularly when those challenges are aggressive or create discomfort.

The techniques in this section comprise the initial approaches to use in virtually any conflicted situation: they are 'first response' skills to bring forward as soon as you sense conflict or defensiveness becoming problematic or as a beginning point in resolving long-standing difficulties.

THINK OF DEFENSIVENESS AND CONFLICT AS A POSITIVE TENSION

Work on mindset prior to experiencing difficulty. Participants rarely try to create problems intentionally. It helps if you and your learners can think of defensiveness and conflict as positive tensions – a natural and inevitable part of skills learning which is full of opportunity – rather than as failures or negative forces (Foreman *et al.* 1996).

USE THE ACCEPTING RESPONSE

Use the accepting response often, particularly when strong feelings (positive or negative) are present (Briggs and Banahan 1979). Also called the 'supportive response' or the 'acknowledging response', the accepting response provides a practical and specific way of:

- accepting non-judgementally what the learner says
- acknowledging the right of the learner to hold their own views and feelings
- valuing the learner's contributions.

This approach is effective because it establishes common ground between facilitator and learner through a shared understanding of the learner's perspective.

The primary characteristic of the accepting response is that it expresses acknowledgement and acceptance of the other person's feelings or ideas and confirms his or her right to have them. Expressing acceptance builds a base for trust. It is not an attempt to help the other person overcome negative feelings or alter ideas with which we disagree. It does not offer agreement or disagreement, attempt to correct misperceptions or offer reassurance. Those steps can come later if they are appropriate. Instead, the accepting response expresses understanding, support and acceptance of where the other person 'is' or how he feels. Acceptance here means acknowledgement and *not* agreement. For example, in response to an outburst of angry words, the accepting response might be:

'I can feel how angry you are; feeling angry is fair enough'
or if someone disagrees strongly:
'Yes, that's clearly another way to look at this – an interesting alternative ...'

Then pause – allow time for the other person to feel accepted. Do not at this time offer help or advice or try to talk the other person into feeling or acting differently. Also guard against hesitating briefly and then going on with 'But ...'.

The acknowledging response helps to establish or re-establish acceptance and therefore trust. The other person will often briefly respond with more of whatever emotion or idea they were expressing. Again employ the accepting response followed by silence. Usually at this point the accepting response will have laid the foundations of a non-defensive atmosphere that enables the parties involved to re-establish common ground, go on with constructive problem solving, correct misperceptions and think through alternatives. We describe the accepting response more fully in the context of doctor–patient communication in our companion volume.

PARAPHRASE

Paraphrase frequently – restate in your own words your perception of the content of the other person's message and/or the feelings that go with it. Paraphrasing is an attempt to verify that your interpretation of the message is the same as the other person's intended meaning. Encourage all involved to paraphrase important parts of the interaction to make sure that everyone understands each other accurately. Work at becoming aware of and confirming unstated assumptions that you think may cause distortions in your own perception or that of others. The accepting response and paraphrasing skills are especially important with cross-cultural groups.

RE-ESTABLISH COMMON GROUND (THE BAKER MODEL)

After acceptance, continue conflict management by returning to a point where there is mutually understood common ground. That common ground may, for example, be an openly discussed and mutually understood definition of the problem. It is usually better to start problem solving and conflict management with a focus on common ground regarding smaller issues of disagreement rather than larger ones, because:

- it is easier to establish common ground and make progress on smaller issues
- such a focus assists all parties to develop a stake in working on tougher issues and reaching resolution.

Stop whenever silences feel noticeably uncomfortable and re-establish what the mutually understood common ground is. Proceed again to try to deal with the conflict when silence feels relatively more comfortable. This tactic also helps prevent escalation from simple disagreement to ego conflict where participants start attacking each other personally. The latter is much more difficult to manage.

REVIEW AND INTENTIONALLY USE GIBB'S STRATEGIES REGARDING SUPPORTIVE AND DEFENSIVE CLIMATES

These behaviours are especially significant when dealing with conflict since some degree of defensiveness is inevitable whenever conflict occurs. A word of caution is necessary here: distinguish carefully between defensiveness and fair defence. Labelling others as defensive can be a way of discounting them and/or their fair defence of their actions. Such discounting in effect gives you and the group inappropriate permission to ignore what is being said or to stop listening altogether.

LEARN TO SAY AND PRACTISE SAYING: 'I'M SORRY' OR 'I WAS WRONG' OR 'I NEVER THOUGHT OF/KNEW THAT; THANKS FOR ENLIGHTENING ME.'

Used sincerely, these simple phrases are remarkably effective.

THINK ABOUT CONFLICT MANAGEMENT AS A HELICAL PROCESS

People tend to view dealing with conflict as a linear process. They expect that once a point is argued or 'won' the conflict regarding that point should be over. Or they assume that once a conflict arises and kicks defensiveness into action, they have reached the 'end of the road' and have a hopeless or at least badly compromised situation on their hands. A more productive choice is to view conflict management, like all communication and learning, as a helical process in which participants have to keep coming back around the spiral, covering the same issues over again at a little higher level, sometimes even backsliding before they can attain satisfactory resolution. The helical model helps us anticipate the course of conflict more realistically when we cover 'old' ground repeatedly or encounter setbacks. The helix encourages both learners and facilitators to keep in mind that real progress is often gradual and requires only that we take one 'next step' at a time on our way up the helix rather than some sort of grand leap. In addition to being a helical process itself, conflict is often part of the helix of learning and change, a precursor to significant gains.

Dealing with tensions that influence learning

One certainty of all experiential learning and especially communication skills work is that strong feelings will feature from time to time. Because communication is so closely bound to self-concept and esteem, feelings from mild frustration to outright anger are likely to accompany the issues of self-confidence, defensiveness and conflict that we have just discussed. Challenging assumptions and asking colleagues to take the risk of trying out new or alternative approaches add another layer of feeling: fear of the unknown, of risk-taking, of making mistakes or failing. These anxieties can prove to be unfounded in a well-facilitated group or one-to-one learning setting but most of us still experience them some of the time. In addition to the material presented above, what techniques can we recommend to facilitators and learners to deal with these tensions?

Much of the discussion that follows focuses on how feelings can help or hinder the learning process and how facilitators can deal with feelings so that communication skills learning is maximized. We make a distinction here between working with feelings in the context of communication skills learning and working in a counselling or group therapy mode. The boundary between group facilitation and therapy is often a thin one. It is not surprising that when doctors or students work in a supportive group environment, they disclose feelings, values and beliefs which can be intense. The question for the facilitator is how far to explore these emotions within the group: can we clarify the boundaries of learning groups?

The emotions that arise may, of course, be unrelated to the communication issues at hand and simply surface in the supportive environment that has been established. In this case, the facilitator has to balance the value and appropriateness to the individual of exploring his emotions here and now during the group session against the importance of continuing with the group's communication learning. Just because emotions have surfaced does not mean the individual necessarily wishes to explore them further; they may not be for public consumption. When feelings are related to the communication problems under discussion, there are still potential dangers of exploring such personal feelings in a group situation without the possibility of long-term support and without the facilitator having the necessary and considerable skills to lead a group therapy session. On the other hand, a skilled facilitator may be able to assist a learner in exploring difficult feelings and enable the whole group to be empathic and collaborative in finding helpful suggestions so that the learning experience is enriched for everybody.

In the discussion that follows, we stress the importance of understanding how feelings and difficulties which lead to tension can influence group learning, explore ways to recognize when this is occurring and provide various strategies for working with the tensions and emotions that emerge. We shall not examine the skills of counselling or therapy which we feel are beyond the remit of most learning groups and certainly of this book.

DISTINGUISHING BETWEEN TYPES OF TENSION

Feelings may emanate from two different kinds of conflict or tension (Miller and Steinberg 1975; Stewart and D'Angelo 1975; Foreman *et al.* 1996):

1 **intrapersonal** (conflict within oneself):
   - issues of confidence and self-esteem
   - anxiety or nervousness

- identification or resonances with past experience
- fear of mistakes, failure or risk taking

2 **interpersonal** (conflict between groups or individuals):
  - content conflict over definitions, interpretations, accuracy
  - basic values conflict over philosophical or ideological differences
  - pseudo conflict over misunderstandings (i.e. no conflict actually exists)
  - simple conflict where one party must lose for the other to win
  - ego conflict where parties attack each other on expertise or competence, personal worth, image, who has power over whom.

Stepping back to determine what kind of conflict or tension might be behind the emotion is a useful first step to dealing with emotions and managing conflict since different kinds of conflict require different management techniques. Ego conflict is rarely, if ever, the starting point. Rather, any one of the other types escalates into ego conflict if the focus shifts from the issue that is at stake to the people who are involved. Since ego conflict is potentially the most devastating, preventing the escalation by shifting discussion immediately away from attacks on a person and back to discussion of issues is useful. This is usually easier to do when you are a third party than when the ego attack is directed at (or coming from) you. When dealing with any difficult emotion – and especially when faced with ego conflict – intentionally use the 'first response' skills for managing conflicted and defended situations described above.

WORKING ON IMPROVING LOW CONFIDENCE OR LOW SELF-ESTEEM

Low confidence or low self-esteem can block learning and change just as increased confidence and self-esteem can enhance them. Lack of confidence or low self-esteem is usually accompanied by anxiety or nervousness which can get in the way of learning, accurate information exchange and competent performance. Paradoxically, low self-esteem and lack of confidence are often the true feelings behind displays of arrogance or overconfidence. While these last two behaviours may be understandable, they are always inappropriate. They draw negative responses from patients and colleagues alike and can yield unfortunate results clinically, such as distorted or omitted information gathering or getting in over your head with respect to treatment or advice.

Some anxiety and lack of confidence are natural and inevitable parts of learning. Time and experience usually resolve the problem. Nonetheless, it is useful for both facilitators and learners to develop skills which help reduce negative effects and increase confidence or self-esteem (Riccardi and Kurtz 1983).

- Give the group (and yourself) licence to talk about such feelings, perhaps by discussing what makes each member uneasy, personal reactions to such feelings, and remedies participants find useful to dispel them.
- During videotape and feedback sessions, reflect on how participants perceive this aspect of one another. Focus on offering descriptive rather than evaluative feedback. Avoid labelling such behaviour as though it were a 'fixed' personality trait, e.g. pinpoint observable behaviours that give the impression of arrogance or anxiety rather than saying 'You're really arrogant [or anxious]'.
- Encourage use of relaxed breathing, muscle relaxation, imaging, yoga, meditation, self-affirmation and other forms of biofeedback and autosuggestion.

- Intentionally use behaviours that make you appear relaxed and confident even if you do not feel that way. Others will then tend to respond to you as though you were confident and relaxed which will, in turn, actually help make you feel so (Mehrabian and Ksionsky 1974; DeVito 1988). Such behaviours include:
  - moving (e.g. gestures, changing posture, shifting in your chair, changes in facial expression) reduces tension and gives others 'permission' to move as well
  - assuming asymmetrical positions in which one side of your body looks different from the other is a simple and effective way to help yourself feel and look more relaxed and confident (e.g. one arm on an armrest and the other in your lap rather than both in your lap)
  - expressing dynamism or responsiveness (e.g. through facial and vocal animation as opposed to flat vocal or rigid facial expression) – dynamism has an added benefit of reflecting how important one individual is to the other (the more responsive I am, the more important you take yourself to be in my eyes)
  - clarifying agendas, sharing your thinking, summarizing and adding structure to the session all tend to increase efficiency and reduce aimless or out-of-sequence questions that appear to reflect lack of confidence.

HANDLING MISTAKES, FAILURE AND RISK-TAKING FEARS

Nobody wants to look foolish. Nobody wants to fail. But everyone will do so in the process of developing communication skills to a professional level. This is an important reason for setting up a supportive climate where learners feel safe to risk and make mistakes. Our discussion of rehearsal and descriptive feedback in Chapters 3 and 5 and the earlier material that we have presented in this chapter describe how to achieve this. Several specific skills are of particular value here:

- emphasize and discuss alternatives for moving ahead rather than trying to come up with a single best approach
- offer opportunities to repeat, to try again
- encourage learners to take 'time out' from an interview in progress and get help from observers when they want to
- think out loud in terms of the helix, e.g. ask learners what 'next steps' they are trying out and only ask that they try those specific steps rather than a perfect performance
- encourage learners to view a perceived mistake or failure as simply one option tried among many
- explain that if mistakes are not happening neither is learning. Frustration can be viewed as an indicator of progress which often immediately precedes a learning breakthrough.

We return again to the study of one attending doctor's bedside teaching rounds which revealed a number of techniques for handling mistakes in small learning groups (Kurtz 1990). Learners reported consistently that these rounds were especially useful, pointing out that the way this attending physician handled mistakes was one of the particular skills that contributed to their learning so much with him. He used mistakes or oversights (his own as well as learners') as a springboard for learning rather than an opportunity for put-downs or criticism. He led learners to conclude for themselves (silently or out loud) that they were wrong rather than saying 'You're wrong' outright and often helped them move toward correcting their mistakes in the process. His techniques for handling wrong answers and other mistakes include:

- asking another more focused question instead of telling learners they're wrong: *'You're thinking fibroids are the problem. But what's causing the liver problems and weight loss?'*
- if conflicts concern opinions rather than right or wrong facts, responding with: *'People differ a lot ...'* or *'My preference on that is ...'*
- refocusing learners' thinking explicitly when they are overlooking important aspects: *'Remember, the objective here is to minimize time in hospital now, because later he'll be in a lot.'*
- after someone admits not knowing what to do, asking other learners for their ideas; if no one knows, inviting learners to guess or going through his own thought process out loud and asking some leading questions
- commenting on his own uncertainty or lack of understanding and sometimes suggesting how he would remedy the shortcoming, thus encouraging students to admit to and remedy their own shortcomings more openly.

Not surprisingly, in these rounds learners freely admitted to their mistakes or lack of knowledge and corrected them on the spot; the attending doctor's techniques left learners free to think and try alternatives rather than defend themselves.

Seeing errors, disagreement and conflict as useful positive tensions and natural parts of participation and learning rather than as indicators of failure, ineptitude or weakness represents a significant shift in perception.

HANDLING DISAGREEMENTS

In an involved group focusing on learning communication skills where everyone is participating, differences of opinion and disagreements are inevitable. What do you do when confronted with disagreements that threaten to escalate into ego conflicts or otherwise block learning or change? Consider the following.

- *Is the conflict 'real'?* To find out, use the acknowledging response, paraphrasing and careful listening to clarify the issues and establish common ground. Often, no further step is required. If necessary, correct distortions and errors of perception. Limit disagreement and discussion about it to one issue at a time.
- *If a 'real' conflict exists,* remind the group of two important mindsets:
  - you can only really decide what is effective when you know what outcomes you are trying to achieve. Ask what goals or outcomes those who are disagreeing have in mind and encourage the group to think about what is effective within that context
  - consensus is often not necessary. Many disagreements can be disarmed simply by pointing out that there is no need for everyone to agree. Since one goal of communication training is for learners to expand their repertoire of skills, consensus may even be counter-productive. Indeed, lack of consensus is often constructive conflict which opens learners up to change. Instead of looking for the 'best' solution or strategy or the 'only' way to do or phrase something, remind learners that the focus is on extending their repertoire.
- *In the case of values conflicts,* agreeing to disagree, and acknowledging this out loud, is usually the only immediate 'solution' possible. In the longer term, influencing by modelling,

by how you act rather than what you say, is useful; so is remaining open to future discussion and enlightenment, which may well lead to changes in your own perspective.

- *If you are the one disagreeing with the rest of the group:*
  - trust the group and be part of it – whether you are facilitator or group member, you have a right to contribute and to equal say
  - respond with: '*Interesting ... my views are different; my offer would be ...*' – value the person with the alternative point of view
  - make your comment a suggestion or alternative and ask the others what they think, i.e. be up front, avoid a hidden agenda
  - if you think the point is very important, say so respectfully: '*This is an important issue for me – I feel strongly about it. Obviously it's not the only way to go but do give it some thought.*'
  - in response to others' comments, use: '*Yes, and ...*' or '*On the other hand ...*' rather than '*Yes, but ...*'
  - relax and stay with supportive rather than defensive behaviours, e.g. offers, suggestions, equality. In other words, avoid escalating to ego conflict.
- *Holding up a mirror to the group.* When you want participants to think about the process of what is happening in the group, say: '*Here's what I see ... What do you think ...?*'. This technique is appropriate both when you are involved in the disagreement yourself and when you are facilitating conflict management as a third party.

DEALING WITH ANGER

The process of exploring mistakes and disagreements opens up consideration of an emotion which accompanies many conflicted or defended situations. Anger (in its greater and lesser forms) seems to create difficulties for most of us regardless of whether the anger is our own, someone else's directed at us or someone else's directed elsewhere that we are merely observing. Understanding anger can help in devising strategies for dealing with it more effectively.

To begin with, anger is a secondary emotion – it does not occur alone but always in conjunction with other 'primary' emotions (Gorden and Burch 1974). For example, we become angry when we are too frustrated or frightened or hurt.

Zeeman's (1976) model of aggression offers an important insight into anger and how people react when they are in conflicted or defended situations, especially when conflicts escalate from relatively benign disagreements into ego conflict. The model suggests that aggression and anger do not follow a consistent linear progression which would increase at predictable increments. Rather, aggression escalates suddenly. For a time, the progression seems to follow along a straight line or one that curves gradually upward. However, at some unpredictable point, the gradually increasing level of aggression leaps up suddenly and exponentially to an altogether different plane. This theory is helpful in understanding what happens to people when anger escalates to verbal (or physical) violence or when one of the more benign types of conflict escalates to ego conflict. A leap may also occur to a different plane altogether wherein the shift is from focus on the problem to focus on the person.

The ideas about anger as a secondary emotion and the model of aggression give us clues about how to deal with anger and conflict:

- regardless of whether it is your own anger or someone else's, respond to it before the 'leap' happens. If you want to control anger or constructively channel the energy it generates, respond to it as a sort of signalling device. When you first sense its presence, focus on putting anger to use; get in touch with it before it escalates and 'leaps'. Think of anger as a message from within that signals you (in time for constructive action): 'Something is wrong here, get in touch with what it is now so you can deal with it'

- if the 'leap' already appears to have happened, taking time out to cool off before trying to reason with each other may help
- focus on the primary emotion beneath the anger, on what the primary emotion is and what is causing it. Work from there rather than focusing on the anger alone.

Anger, fear, frustration, sensitivity, giddiness, excitement – some kind of emotion almost always accompanies conflict. We have found one final suggestion for dealing with emotions particularly important to remember: regardless of their negative or positive qualities, emotions are natural and potentially useful because they help us to focus on the experiences with which they are associated. Emotions heighten our ability to engage, learn and change. Perhaps that is why emotions, and the conflicts that give rise to them, are so commonly part of our learning experience.

Dealing with specific difficulties: putting the skills into practice

In this chapter, we have described several skills and strategies for effective facilitation in the face of challenging situations. The following are two examples of difficulties that frequently arise in group learning and demonstrate how a facilitator might combine these skills in practice.

Example 1: responding to judgemental or unsafe feedback from a group member
This example explores how to respond when a group member (who may, in an unfocused moment, be the facilitator!) gives unsafe or judgemental feedback. To maximize learning both for the person receiving feedback and the rest of the group, a necessary precondition is a supportive environment in which criticism can be accepted and assimilated. Judgemental or aggressive feedback creates defensiveness and diminishes learning. For the facilitator this creates two challenges:

1 how to counter the judgemental criticism without being judgemental yourself and thereby creating further defensiveness
2 how, while rushing in to rescue the person receiving feedback, to defuse the aggressive criticism and at the same time support the person who gave it.

THE UNDESIRED OUTCOME

Group member: *'That was awful. You didn't pick up any of the patient's cues. It was terrible.'*
Translation: the interview was rubbish and so probably are you

Facilitator (rescuing the person receiving feedback): *'Hold on, you can't give that sort of feedback. Don't be so aggressive. How do you think that makes John feel?'*
Translation: the feedback was rubbish and so probably are you

Another group member (rescuing the first): *'But I agree with Dave, it was awful.'*
Translation: your intervention is rubbish and so probably are you

Facilitator (now defensive and still trying to rescue John): *'John, how did Dave's feedback make you feel?'*
Translation: help, I'm now feeling defensive and need rescuing

John (being brave and rescuing Dave): *'I didn't mind at all. Dave always says a spade's a spade – he can't help being a nerd!'*
Translation: I'm now feeling even worse what with all this attention on how awful I must feel

Facilitator looks for hole in floor.

A BETTER PLAN

- **Separate the message (what the feedback said) from the delivery (how it was said), i.e. the content from the process.** Often the participant is making a good point but in the wrong way. It is easy to overlook good content while tackling poor process.
- **Model non-judgemental, descriptive feedback.** Instead of fighting judgement with judgement, model the appropriate descriptive skills.
- **Support and value both the person doing the interview and the participant giving the feedback.** Both potentially require rescuing from a difficult situation: taking sides or highlighting someone's need for protection by intervening too heavily may make matters worse.

OPTIONS FOR PUTTING THE PLAN INTO ACTION

- **Rather than confront, encourage participants to use descriptive feedback**. In place of *'That was very difficult feedback'*, move the process forward with:

  'When you say awful, what did you see that didn't work for you?'

  This is non-confrontational modelling and helps demonstrate what you want without confronting behaviour directly. Appropriate descriptive feedback is obtained without denigrating the participant; the participant's feedback is acknowledged; the person receiving feedback does not have his discomfiture made even more obvious; and both people are valued.
- **Signpost how descriptive feedback would help the group**. A slightly different approach is to signpost to the participant why you are suggesting a change in their feedback:

  'That's an interesting point. Could we look specifically at what you saw that didn't seem to work; not so much whether it was good or bad, but describing exactly what cues you saw that you felt were important? Then we can all look at what we might want to achieve here and think of ways of doing it.'

  This values the participant while gently explaining the need for more specific and descriptive feedback rather than general and evaluative comments. And it refocuses attention on the outcomes the doctor and patient are trying to achieve, thus opening the way for deciding what approaches might be most effective in achieving those outcomes.
- **Own your own thoughts**. If the feedback is obviously judgemental, smile, grimace, clutch your hands to your heart and say:

  'Hey, that hurt, did anyone else feel that?'

i.e. just react as a member of the group and check your reactions with the other group members. This is a humorous approach at defusing the situation and works if the group is well formed and the atmosphere is trusting and supportive. Follow up with a big smile and:

'Dave, quickly rephrase that before John kills himself!'

- **Rephrase it yourself without fuss**.

  'Good comment. Can I just rephrase it to make it easier to work with? "On several occasions the patient seemed to give out cues that she was worried." Is that what you saw, Dave?'

  This quickly adjusts the feedback without undue emphasis on the giver or receiver.
- **Check out with the recipient and the group**. Signpost why you are asking first before checking out the feedback with the recipient:

  'That's an important point, Dave. I wonder about the style of feedback, not what you said which I think is very interesting but how you said it. I was wondering if we were veering away from the ground rules we looked at earlier or if it's still OK for the group. Could I just check that out with John and the rest of the group?'

  Try not to label the behaviour yourself but get the group to label and sort out what they would prefer. If not, say:

  'If it were me, it would make me defensive. What do you think?'

  (still do not label the comments as aggressive, etc.).
- **Look at feedback in the group in general**. Often it can be preferable not to point the finger of blame directly at one person.

  'Could we step back for a moment and look at the process? How are we doing here on feedback – is it working? Is there anything we can improve on?'

- **Or hold up a mirror to the group**.

  'Here's what I see happening. It looks like we are focusing more on the negative – is that what you want to do?'

  or

  'We're tending to open with negative comments, for example ...'

  and then quote in the tone in which they were said without attributing them necessarily to a person or labelling them as tough to take.

  'Is that OK for you? Is that a constructive way to proceed?'

  Link interaction in the learning group with interaction in the consultation. Our comments to each other are like the comments we make to patients, always requiring that we pay attention to their effect on the recipient.
- **If you have made the mistake yourself of giving judgemental feedback, catch yourself and say so out loud**.

  'Wait a minute – I'm sorry, that was not useful feedback. Let me step back and try that again ...'

  No one remains perfectly focused one hundred per cent of the time. Publicly admitting to and remedying your own mistakes corrects the error, models how you use your mistakes as a springboard for learning and encourages learners to admit to, and remedy, their own shortcomings more openly.

Example 2: dealing with unsupportive or disruptive group members
In this second example, we look at the difficulty of dealing with unsupportive or disruptive group members. This is a challenging problem for the facilitator that can take many different forms, including:

- a direct challenge to the leadership (overt aggression)
- unsupportive or critical behaviour to other group members
- refusal to buy in to the process (will not role play, show tapes, give feedback)
- overconfidence or competitiveness leading to overcontribution or arrogance
- silence or sullenness, non-contribution (passive aggression)
- sabotage, disruption of the process or structure of the group (deliberate or not deliberate)
- the out-of-control group.

STRATEGIES FOR DEALING WITH THESE SITUATIONS

Check your mindset, remembering that:

- conflict or difficult behaviour is healthy and normal
- all difficult behaviour is communicating something
- the 'difficult' person may be saying something that everyone else in the group is thinking; what looks like difficult behaviour may in fact be brave behaviour
- separate the content and the process of the message and consider the meanings of both.

Begin with the 'first response' skills that we have described above for use in any conflicted or defended situations, especially where the behaviour is overt and direct:

- use the accepting response
- paraphrase
- re-establish common ground (the Baker model)
- review and intentionally use Gibb's strategies regarding defensive and supportive climates
- learn to say and practise saying: 'I'm sorry' or 'I was wrong' or 'I never thought of/knew that; thanks for enlightening me'.

However, in many of the situations that we have listed above, the difficult or disruptive behaviour is not an overt challenge and remains an unspoken and occasionally unrecognized issue within the group. If, for instance, the group members are all talking at once rather than listening to each other's comments or are way off task, or if one member of the group is sullen or over-contributing, the facilitator has to decide how to return the group to more appropriate working patterns or whether to bring the behaviour in question out into the open for overt discussion.
Any of the following additional approaches can be useful:

- **Share the facilitator's dilemma verbally**. Checking out the facilitator's dilemma with the group is an overt and involving method of dealing with difficulties. 'Holding up a mirror' is one way to achieve this:

  'I'd like to call time out and look at what is happening in the group … Here's what I see happening.

I see some of the group talking most of the time and others who have yet to speak. What do you think? Are you happy with that?

- **Own your own feelings and check with the group**. Speak for yourself rather than for the group:

  'I feel uncomfortable at the moment with the way we're tackling things today. I sense myself becoming increasingly defensive and concerned. Can I check out what's happening and how you are all feeling about it?'

- **Reflect the group back to its ground rules**. Reflect the group back to previously established ground rules and ask if they are abiding by them. Check out if they are comfortable with the process as it stands.
- **Reflect the group back to the agenda for this feedback session**. Re-establish direction and task by seeing if the group is still working constructively on their original agenda.
- **Break to a 'round' re the group's current task**. Asking each group member to state their ideas in a round about the issue that is the group's current focus of discussion encourages each member to contribute and re-establishes a climate of listening and respect. It is especially helpful if one member is overcontributing. Saying *'That's interesting. Let's see what everybody else thinks …'* and going round the group values the contributor while still allowing the rest of the group in.
- **Break to a 'round' re feelings**. This enables all members to contribute their feelings about the group process or task without singling one individual out (such as the non-contributor).
- **Break to a pairs listening exercise re the group's current task**. Rather than concentrating on the difficult behaviour that has arisen, a listening exercise where pairs of learners discuss the issue the group is working on encourages participation by everyone and enables learners to re-establish appropriate patterns of listening and contribution without highlighting the difficulty overtly. Such exercises also break things up, give the leader time to think and reflect and make the group process more dynamic. Ideas discussed in the pairs can then be shared with the group as a whole.
- **Break to a pairs listening exercise re process**. A pairs listening exercise can also be used to enable the group to address the group dynamics which are causing difficulties. This enables a change of direction and allows time for reflection.
- **Singling people out**. Confronting an individual member of the group is a high-risk strategy. The facilitator must choose carefully between ignoring the behaviour, attempting to tackle the issue within the group setting or waiting to discuss the issue later in private. Asking *'How are you, Richard?'* to the sullen member within the group can lead to a clearer understanding of the difficulty (which could be tiredness, other concerns from outside the room or anxiety or discomfort about the teaching method). However, it may disrupt the learning of the group or force the learner to expose a private issue to the group against his better judgement and wishes. If there is any doubt, it is safer to wait and have a conversation in private, especially if the group is not well established and if individuals are not well known to you as yet.

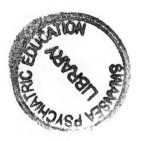

7

Running a session: introducing research and theory: expanding and consolidating learning

Introduction

In this chapter we explore how to introduce research evidence and communication theory into experiential learning and how to expand and consolidate discussion so that it results in greater understanding and skill development.

As we discussed in Chapters 5 and 6, the facilitator has many responsibilities in communication skills teaching related to group *process*. These include:

- developing and maintaining a supportive environment
- ensuring descriptive and non-judgemental feedback
- facilitating the group's discussion
- keeping the group focused and moving forward
- summarizing learning
- dealing with defensiveness and conflict constructively.

We also described how the facilitator has equally important responsibilities with respect to the *content* of the learning session:

- ensuring that each learner receives constructive feedback about individual consultations and assistance in *personal skill development*
- *expanding discussion and learning* by encouraging the sharing and exploration of personal experience and ideas and by periodically *consolidating what the group has learned* from discussion

- deepening discussion and learning by *introducing relevant communication concepts, principles and research evidence* – balancing personal ideas and experiential learning with broader perspectives from the literature.

It is the facilitator's task to introduce selected and appropriate content into experiential learning at just the point where it will most help learners and complement their self-exploration. In this chapter we explore practical ways to achieve this.

If facilitators are to accomplish this task, they must have information about communication research and theory at their fingertips. As a teacher, it is not sufficient to know only 'how' to teach communication skills; understanding 'what' to teach – and how to present the 'what' in ways that learners can make use of it – is equally important. Our companion book, *Skills for Communicating with Patients*, is designed to provide programme directors and facilitators with the information that they require to teach this subject with confidence.

While learners will benefit greatly from reading this material for themselves, facilitators still bear responsibility for introducing concepts, principles and research from the literature at opportune moments during experiential sessions. When material is introduced in context and applied directly to learners' current discussion, it is more likely to influence learning and skill development. As the course progresses and their knowledge and skills increase, learners can be invited to assist with this responsibility. The tennis analogy is useful again – it helps if you read about how to improve your game but it helps more if following your reading, you work with an experienced coach who can discuss what you have read and help you relate it at appropriate moments to what you are doing on the court.

In this chapter we provide an overview of methods and techniques which help to:

- introduce relevant didactic teaching into experiential learning
- expand and consolidate experience and discussion.

We then discuss:

- specific and practical suggestions for implementing these two tasks in relation to:
  - all five tasks of the *Calgary–Cambridge observation guide*
  - selected communication issues.

This chapter provides a direct link between this book on how to teach and learn communication skills and our companion volume which presents the theory and research evidence behind the skills. We encourage readers to use our companion volume in conjunction with this chapter. To make that task easier, both this chapter's suggestions regarding the five consultation tasks and our companion volume follow the same structure as the *Calgary–Cambridge observation guide*.

An overview: how to introduce didactic teaching and expand and consolidate experience and discussion

Balancing experiential learning and opportunistic teaching is a delicate task requiring frequent checking of learners' educational needs. Although in this chapter we provide a broad range of suggestions for facilitators to use, we stress that it is only necessary to introduce one or two of these ideas into any one session. Facilitators need to keep the principles of adult learning constantly in mind and work primarily from learners' agendas rather than their own teaching agenda. Awareness of the danger of 'overteaching' is very important.

Introducing communication concepts, principles and research opportunistically

Many opportunities arise for a facilitator to introduce important points from theory or research to illuminate a particular area of the consultation that the group is exploring. This can be achieved in two ways:

1 ask permission from the group to generalize away from discussing the specific consultation under review into a mini-lecture about relevant communication concepts, principles or research. Float this as an offer to see if this input seems appropriate to participants and find out what they already know. For example: *'Do you know the research evidence that supports the value of understanding the patient's perspective of their illness?'* followed by *'Would you like to know more?'* If participants are interested, proceed with the mini-lecture
2 offer learners the opportunity to bring in relevant theory or research that they can contribute themselves. If anyone already knows some of the literature, ask if they would like to tell the group about it or begin the mini-lecture. You or other participants can then offer additional detail or further cognitive material.

Take care with either approach that the mini-lecture is brief and that you and the group return afterwards to more learner-centred, experiential methods of discussion, observation or rehearsal. For example, 'return the ball' to the learner or the group by asking if the material has been helpful and then deliberately sit back so they can continue with their discussion of the interview in question. Keep checking the balance between how much you as facilitator are talking and how much the group is contributing. By far the greatest proportion of time should go to the learners and their practice, observation and discussion.

Expanding and consolidating experience and discussion

As the session progresses, opportunities will also present themselves where it might help learners to move away from the specific material in the interview to expand and consolidate their learning. Techniques include:

- methods which engage learners and add depth to discussion
- further ways to use role play
- additional approaches to using videotape
- identifying and working with the thoughts and feelings of the patient and the doctor
- methods which summarize learning.

These techniques enable us to move beyond superficial thinking and discussion and deepen experiential learning. They enable us to pull together the ideas and skills that arise in experiential learning into something meaningful and memorable. They engage learners and add depth to both experience and discussion. They provide a useful counterpoint to the interview and move learners forward in their skill development. Once more, these techniques need careful introduction. For example, the facilitator might say:

'Would it be helpful here to generalize away from the interview we are watching and look at the ways which we each use to ask patients about their own ideas and concerns? ... Let's brainstorm the different phrases we have found that work. What are the advantages of each? What are we trying to achieve? ... OK, let's role play a few and see how they feel in practice.'

Again, returning to the interview afterwards is vital:

'Harry, do any of those thoughts help with the situation you were in at the beginning of your interview? Has it given you any ideas you would like to practise?'

METHODS WHICH ENGAGE THE LEARNER AND ADD DEPTH TO DISCUSSION

The following techniques can all help to make learning more dynamic and allow the facilitator to encourage exploration and discussion of a particular skill or part of the consultation:

- rounds, where each member is encouraged to contribute
- pairs or trios exercises
- brainstorming
- flip-charting and recording
- encouraging use of the *Calgary–Cambridge observation guide*
- responding and questioning techniques.

Sometimes group work or exchanges with individual learners can become dull or 'get stuck' or the facilitator loses his way. One or more of the group can become silent, non-contributory, challenging to the facilitator or overdominant; or the discussion fails because it is too vague or superficial. Using any of the above techniques can motivate learners to focus on the concrete, delve beyond the superficial, re-engage, move on and learn – a key factor is the adept use of the responding and questioning techniques which we presented in Chapter 6.

USING ROLE PLAY TO FACILITATE REHEARSAL

We have already discussed the importance of rehearsal in learners' skill development. In particular, we have discussed the value of simulated patients in allowing learners to rehearse skills repeatedly within experiential sessions. We have also explored the value of a group member taking the role of the patient who cannot be present during the teaching session when watching pre-recorded video tapes. Other ways to use role play include:

- mini-role play to rehearse specific phrasing, for example to rehearse phrases to elicit patients' ideas and concerns
- prepared role play in which the learners are given a role as doctor or patient with a specific purpose, for example breaking bad news
- reverse role play is particularly useful if a learner brings an actual case to the group which he would like help with (i.e. the doctor bringing the case plays the patient's role)
- a 'bad' role play followed by a 'good' role play – it breaks the ice and can also help reluctant role players to try the method
- non-medical role play is sometimes helpful and less threatening to the performing doctor or the student lacking clinical experience.

If learners are reluctant to try role playing, it is helpful to discover what the blocks to the method are and to accept the learners' feelings. Gentle but firm encouragement, explaining the theories behind role play or allowing members of the group to suggest phrases first before they try them out with the patient, can help to overcome blocks. Engage willing volunteers first.

OTHER WAYS TO USE VIDEOTAPE

We described the value of video recordings in Chapters 3 and 4. Additional ways to use the tape include:

- using the tape to look specifically at particular skills, e.g. non-verbal behaviour or picking up cues
- playing the video recording with the sound turned off
- 'freeze-framing' a particular moment on the tape
- replaying the same segment of the consultation from several videotapes (e.g. initiation).

IDENTIFYING AND EXPLORING THOUGHTS AND FEELINGS OF BOTH THE PATIENT AND THE DOCTOR

Encouraging learners to sink themselves into the role of the patient often helps to provide insights into how the patient may be feeling and may help doctors to be more patient centred. Asking real patients to come and tell their stories, for example a patient with an illicit drug problem or a bereaved patient or a 'panel' of parents looking after seriously ill children, also allows a group of learners to deepen their understanding. Throughout this book we have encouraged an outcome-based approach to helping learners to look at the appropriate use of communication skills. It can be helpful to explore learners' feelings and thoughts first before looking at what they are trying to achieve and how they might get there. Doing so allows attitudes and skills to be explored hand in hand.

METHODS OF SUMMARIZING LEARNING

Summarizing to reinforce and help learners to structure and remember what they have learned is important. Summarizing exercises include:

- asking learners to write down or flip chart what they have learned
- doing a 'round' of what learners will take away from the teaching session
- using the guide to summarize lessons learned during the session and 'next steps'.

Pattern recognition*

Deciding on which teaching method or piece of research or theory to introduce into any experiential session is not necessarily easy. Fortunately, most problems for learners fall into categories that facilitators soon begin to recognize: common patterns occur commonly, just

* We are grateful to Tony Pearson for suggesting this concept.

like the problems patients present to the doctor! Recognizing that there is a pattern to these problems is helpful as the facilitator can then anticipate patterns and plan accordingly.

In our experience, some of the common problem patterns are as follows:

- the learner does not discover all the issues or problems the patient wishes to discuss, i.e. why the patient has come today
- the learner does not listen, usually due to not asking good, open-ended questions initially or interrupting with closed questions
- the learner does not elicit the patient's ideas, concerns, expectations and feelings or establish a collaborative relationship, and instead takes a doctor-centred position throughout the interview
- the learner develops little rapport or is not responsive to the patient
- the learner misses important cues from the patient
- the learner obtains an inaccurate or incomplete clinical history because of failure to get the balance right between open and closed questions, to summarize and check or to share thinking
- the learner forgets to find out what the patient already knows before giving an explanation
- the learner gives too much information at once and uses jargon
- the learner fails to negotiate with the patient or to check that the patient is agreeable to the plan
- the learner makes inadequate follow-up or safety-netting arrangements.

Useful questions to ask yourself, as the facilitator, as you are watching any consultation are:

- can I recognize any patterns here?
- have I seen this problem before?
- how might the learner who performed the consultation be feeling?
- how might the 'patient' be feeling?
- what does the group already know?
- how could I use this material as a springboard for further learning?
- when would be the best time to do it?
- what area of the consultation or what research and theory would be relevant to focus on here?
- do I have the knowledge?
- do any of the learners have the knowledge?
- is the overall balance between experiential work and didactic material from the literature right for the group?
- do I have an *aide-mémoire*/handout for the group that fits here?

Practical suggestions for introducing theory and research evidence and consolidating learning

We turn now to practical examples of how to introduce theory and research evidence into experiential learning and how to expand and consolidate discussion. Although we present them here in relation to the order of structure and skills in the *Calgary–Cambridge observation guide,* these suggestions can be introduced in any sequence that might help learners during a teaching session on any part of the consultation. To highlight the various techniques that can be used, we have chosen examples concerning areas from each section of the consultation where learners commonly experience difficulties.

Initiating the session

Problems we see commonly in this section of the consultation relate to:

- preparation before the patient comes in
- listening attentively without interrupting at the beginning of the interview
- discovering all the issues or problems the patient wishes to discuss
- setting the agenda for the rest of the interview.

PREPARATION

Focusing attention. So many consultations get off to a bad start because of uncertainties at the beginning of the consultation; for example, not being sure if you have the right patient, not clarifying whether this is a new patient or someone you have met before or not having the results of tests or the specialist's or family physician's letter to hand. Many of these uncertainties can be avoided by a few moments of focused attention and preparation for the interview. **Open discussion** of how doctors use records and computers before the patient is seen can help exploration of these issues of preparation.

ESTABLISHING INITIAL RAPPORT

Using medical records and computers. Looking at how using medical records and computers during the consultation can affect learners' non-verbal communication and at the messages that this imparts to the patient underscores the value of preparation and of putting the records to one side. **Role plays** of opening a simple consultation while flicking through the records and, alternatively, while giving good eye-contact can be particularly instructive, especially when viewed from the perspective of the patient. How non-verbal messages override verbal ones can be demonstrated and the **appropriate research findings offered**.

IDENTIFYING THE ISSUES AND PROBLEMS THE PATIENT WANTS TO DISCUSS

Often the group's discussion centres around not quite knowing or having an incomplete understanding of why the patient has really come. This is equally true for specialist and primary care settings.

The opening question. An excellent place to start looking at this problem is the opening question. Take the pressure off individual learners by **brainstorming** the favourite opening questions that group members routinely use. **Produce a list** and **invite discussion** about how these different questions can subtly change the type of response that the patient gives. Encourage the group to keep in mind that one of the main aims at the beginning of the consultation is to try to discover all the issues and problems the patient wishes to discuss. To accomplish this, prompt learners to ask themselves routinely *'Do I now know why this patient wants to see me?'*.

Listening. The fact that listening is not 'doing nothing' can be picked up in virtually every consultation whether or not good listening skills are demonstrated. If the interviewer shows effective listening skills, it is helpful not just to acknowledge this but to explore exactly what she is doing, to show that she is not 'just sitting there'. **Analyse** the components of listening and **flip chart the behaviours demonstrated**. For example:

- verbal facilitation: um, yes, go on, ah ha
- non-verbal facilitation: position, posture, eye contact, facial expression, animation, tone of voice
- wait-time: length of pause before asking follow-up questions.

Provide evidence from Beckman and Frankel (1984) about the effect of interruptions of the patient's opening statement. Try different openings and techniques of attentive listening using **role play or rehearsing with simulated patients**. If learners are having difficulty with wait-time or find it unnatural, ask if you (or another learner) can sit behind the learner in the role play and **put a hand on her shoulder** as soon as she starts to respond; release it when you yourself would feel the need to ask another question.

Screening and agenda setting. Screening and agenda setting are frequently keys to efficiency in the consultation. Because of the tension between listening and screening in the initiation phase of the interview, we have found it particularly important that the introduction of this task be carefully timed. Doctors like 'doing something' and since screening is an active process it holds many attractions for them. However, there is a real danger that listening, one of the most important skills, might lose out to screening.

It is most profitable to explore the concept of screening with learners when it is on their agenda. Introduce the idea of screening when a related issue is raised by one of the group members ('I'm not sure I know why she came today; there seems to be something else on her mind') or when a second complaint arises late in the interview ('There is one other thing doctor, my leg has turned blue this week'). **Pose the question to the group** 'How did you know the problem you focused on during the history was the only problem on the patient's mind?'. This can lead into a discussion of how easy it is to make assumptions about what the patient wants to discuss.

Suggest that it might be worthwhile **generalizing away** from a learner's specific consultation to consider the problem of late-arising complaints. If you have a list of group members' learning needs which includes problems with endings and time management, **refer back to learners' needs. Provide evidence** that patients often have more than one concern to discuss and that the order in which they present them is not related to their importance (Beckman and Frankel 1984).

Try **mini-role plays** of the exact words that would help to screen the whole of the patient's agenda so that participants have a chance to discover alternative phrasing they would feel comfortable with in practice.

Looking at a following consultation provides an excellent opportunity for exploring the principles of agenda setting. Comparing new and follow-up consultations is useful as they have much in common. **Ask what difficulties learners have experienced** at the beginning of a follow-up visit. This often reveals a set of problems concerning how to start the consultation when you think you already know the reason for the patient's attendance.

Asking for suggestions about how to overcome these problems should help the group to construct a plan that acknowledges the previous consultation and the doctor's assumed agenda, but allows the patient and the doctor to add new agenda items too:

'Am I right in thinking you've come for a check on your angina today?'
'Yes, that's right doctor.'
'Angina ... Was there anything else you wanted to talk about today?'
'No, that's all, just the angina.'
'Good, ... and I'd just like to check the blood tests with you that you had done a couple of weeks ago.'
'Right, ... Tell me how things have been since we last met.'

Offer the communication principle of establishing mutually understood common ground (Baker 1955) and its importance in review appointments.

Comparing the beginnings of several learners' consultations, exploring how each group member performs up until the first closed question is asked, and then **analysing** the effectiveness of the skills used in terms of outcome is a useful approach. (This is easier if you are using videotapes.)

Another good way of looking at the skills of initiation in a non-threatening way is to ask someone to **role play as badly as possible** the beginning of the consultation. Encourage them to have fun with it. Ask one of the group to role play a patient and give them a simple scenario such as a sore throat. Get the doctor to play the scene as they would hope *not* to in reality. Ask the others in the group to see if they can do worse. Draw out the negative skill areas and produce a list of positive alternatives.

Gathering information

Common problems which we encounter in this part of the consultation are:

- underdeveloped skills in using open questions, moving to closed questioning too soon and getting the balance wrong between open and closed questions
- taking an inadequate clinical history
- omitting to discover the patient's perspective
- not providing structure in the consultation.

EXPLORATION OF PROBLEMS

The importance of question style to information gathering. The issue of questioning style comes up frequently. The group's discussion often centres around a feeling that a line of questioning did not get them very far, that they did not discover the best approach to guide them smoothly through the consultation. Repeatedly, we see a group member moving quickly to explore a particular hypothesis with closed questions, only to come up with incomplete information or lose his way. Once the group has managed to identify that this is a problem area, introduce exercises to look at the range of different questioning methods that are available to help learners obtain the information they need more efficiently and accurately.

Learners are not always entirely sure what constitutes an open or closed question; the following is a useful method of exploring this difficulty. **Ask the group's permission to generalize away from the specific** and **get the group to ask you, the facilitator, questions about a non-medical subject** with first closed questions and then open questions:

- give the group a non-medical subject to ask you questions about, e.g. your holidays, your car, your children
- ask them to try out only closed questions and see what information they obtain
- then try open questions/statements and discuss the differences and the timing of open and closed questions in information gathering.

Follow with the same exercise, but this time choose a medical topic, for example your headaches. **Discuss** the advantages of the open approach at the beginning of the consultation and how it helps the learner to listen accurately, lessening the need to be continually thinking of the next question to ask the patient. **Explain** how helpful open questions are if the questioner has limited medical knowledge or no idea about a topic. **Explain** how closed questions are vital when trying to clarify important points of the history and how counter-productive they are if used too early in the history-taking process.

In discussions about questioning, include the value of sharing with patients the rationale for asking particular questions: *'Sometimes, tiredness can be caused by stress. I was wondering if you felt that might be true for you, whether you were under a lot of stress at present?'*. Comparison with *'Are you under a lot of stress at present?'* can reveal the value of sharing your reasoning so that patients do not make false assumptions about your motives, e.g. 'He thinks I'm just neurotic'.

UNDERSTANDING THE PATIENT'S PERSPECTIVE

At some point in the group process it is valuable to ask the learners' permission to **generalize away from the specific issue** and provide a **mini-lecture** on the disease–illness model (McWhinney 1989). This is such an important topic that it more than repays time taken to explain the concept thoroughly: such teaching appears to be greeted by a sudden flash of understanding from at least some of the participants. **Asking learners to sink themselves into the role of a patient** with chest pain, and then asking each of them to share their ideas, concerns and feelings as well as their expectations for the consultation, will result in a number of different belief frameworks about chest pain which the group can then discuss in terms of the importance of not making assumptions about what patients think and believe. **Provide the research evidence** regarding patient beliefs, concerns and expectations and their links to health outcomes and compliance issues.

Specific phrasing of questions about ideas, concerns and expectations. An excellent way to explore the patient's perspective and some of the issues involved in eliciting it is to look at the phrasing of direct questions that ask patients for their ideas and concerns. Bring out the difficulties of phrasing such questions so that both doctor and patient feel comfortable. **Brainstorm** the approaches that the group finds useful. **Produce two separate lists** of possible phrases for ideas and concerns. Try a similar exercise for exploring the patient's expectations for the consultation. Learners often find this the most difficult of the questions about the patient's perspective to ask without appearing either condescending or lacking in knowledge themselves. **Practising exact phrases** can be a very helpful exercise. Try **experimenting using role play** at which point in the information gathering part of the consultation it is most effective to elicit the patient's ideas and concerns.

Sharing why you are asking the patient for their ideas. Often the issue arises from the participants that the patient may not be comfortable with being asked for their views and might respond with 'you're the doctor' type comments. This provides an opportunity for learners to **role play** their replies and talk with the patient about why it is helpful to know what their ideas are.

Feelings. Because this is an area which learners have often been taught to avoid at medical school, you particularly need to **practise** ways of eliciting the patient's feelings so that learners can become confident and relaxed with those skills. Again, **brainstorming, listing on a flip chart or blackboard and discussing** the value of the various ways learners can elicit patients' feelings is a good entry point to this area.

Providing structure to the consultation

Summarizing and signposting are two of the most underused yet most valuable of all communication skills. They are ready-made answers to the very genuine problems of feeling disorganized or out of control that learners identify when experimenting with a patient-centred, collaborative communication style and a more open approach to questioning.

Internal summary and signposting. Summarizing and signposting are ideal subjects with which to **introduce some of the five principles of effective communication** (see Chapter 2) such as *'ensuring an interaction rather than a direct transmission process'* and *'reducing uncertainty'*.

Use **role play** to give participants an opportunity to practise the phrasing of summarizing. **Discuss**:

- how to make a précis of what has been said
- how to signpost your summary
- how to check with the patient that you got it right.

Building the relationship

Some of the skills that give learners problems in the area of relationship building are:

- demonstrating appropriate non-verbal behaviour
- picking up cues
- demonstrating empathy
- involving the patient.

Non-verbal communication

The importance of demonstrating appropriate non-verbal behaviour. While reviewing a consultation, **focus specific attention** on the details of non-verbal behaviour and remind learners to **give**

detailed descriptive feedback. Learners often make points that are vague or general. For example, if someone says, *'You were really sympathetic with that patient'*, request (or model) more specific and concrete feedback regarding the non-verbal behaviour they observed which demonstrated rapport or responsiveness:

'I saw you lean forward towards the patient at that point, Jane. You were careful to maintain eye contact, and she then relaxed and sat back in her chair ... What do you think?'

'Yes, I wasn't sure whether I was too close to her, but it did seem to help her relax and look more comfortable.'

Flip chart and **clarify** non-verbal behaviours that demonstrate particular attitudes or feelings. The list for responsiveness, for example, might include expressive use of the voice, facial expression which varies to match what the patient is saying, forward lean, etc. This technique provides an easy entry into 'let's look and see what happens next', that is, paying attention to the *effect* of the non-verbal behaviour. The facilitator can then move on to suggestions for improvement and encourage rehearsal of those suggestions. Watching a tape without the sound turned up can be a useful and light-hearted way of exploring non-verbal behaviour and its effects on patients.

Use a **mini-lecture** to introduce the theoretical and the research evidence which supports the use of effective non-verbal behaviour in the consultation; for example, that non-verbal communication is an inevitable occurrence and not always under our voluntary control; it is the channel most responsible for conveying our attitudes, emotions and affect. Quote, for example, Goldberg *et al.'s* (1983) study showing that doctors who establish eye contact are more likely to detect emotional distress in their patients. Discuss how non-verbal messages tend to override what we actually say to patients if our non-verbal and verbal messages contradict each other.

Picking up patients' non-verbal cues. Picking up patients' non-verbal cues, decoding them and, most importantly, checking that our interpretations are correct are crucial to understanding patients' emotions and feelings.

A useful exercise is to **stop the tape** whenever the patient 'drops' a significant non-verbal cue (Gask *et al.* 1991) and look at what the patient might be thinking, feeling or trying to say. The other alternative is to use a 'trigger' or prepared tape. **Describe** and **analyse** the non-verbal cues given by the patient; **discuss** their possible meaning; **rehearse** precise phrases to use when checking them out with the patient and how to incorporate and use that information in the consultation:

'... so we've noticed that the patient looked sad at that point ... Any ideas about what that might be about? ... How would you reflect that back to the patient to check out your interpretation ...? ... Now let's see how we can link that in with what the patient has already told us in a helpful way ... or use that information to discover more about her concerns.'

This gives the group an opportunity for further exploration and rehearsal of skills. **Ask the role player or simulated patient** to illuminate the discussion by telling the group how they are feeling and how acceptable and helpful they find the group's suggestions. This approach may help the learner who finds it difficult to be patient centred.

Role playing telephone consultations when the learner is deprived of many non-verbal cues facilitates discussion of the importance of checking out the doctor's assumptions and provides more opportunities for rehearsal of skills. Try the technique of sitting the doctor and the patient back to back with a telephone each.

Exploring the question 'What prevents the doctor from picking up the patient's cues?' may uncover a number of concerns for learners which are both conscious and unconscious. The facilitator needs to be sensitive when using this exercise. Try a **paired listening exercise** first and then get the group to feed back their blocks and **flip chart** the difficulties. The list might contain the following:

- fear of the patient unloading all their problems onto me
- no time
- feeling out of control
- being uncertain about the clinical content of the consultation
- telephone interruptions
- not liking the patient
- feeling too close to the patient.

Take enough time to explore these blocks and see what strategies and solutions the group can find to help each other.

DEVELOPING RAPPORT

Empathy. Empathy is not a word that is well understood by doctors. It is often confused with sympathy. It is well worth **exploring the group's definitions** of the term, summarizing them and working out a common definition. Learners may say that they cannot fully appreciate their patient's position as they have not experienced it themselves. **Explain** that it is not necessary to have had direct experience of a problem in order to be empathic. It may be enough to show the patient that you are being sensitive and are attempting to put yourself in their position and understand how they view the world. **Work out exact phrases** which demonstrate empathy in specific situations. You may need to give examples to **demonstrate** that one key to making empathic statements is linking the 'I' of the doctor and the 'you' of the patient.

INVOLVING THE PATIENT

One of the most rewarding skills to teach learners is how to involve the patient in the process of the consultation. In our experience this is not a strategy which is commonly taught. We frequently see a friendly and empathic style used in the information-gathering part of the consultation but not much effort to involve the patient as a partner in the process. Learners frequently use an even more doctor-centred and somewhat authoritarian approach to patients in relation to giving a diagnosis and explanation and planning.

Sharing of thoughts. Give a **mini-lecture** on the principle that effective communication prevents uncertainty. Encourage the group to **list** phrases which allow learners to share their thoughts out loud at appropriate points in the consultation. Check how learners feel about this type of collaborative approach. **Discuss** any difficulties, for example concern with loss of professionalism, inappropriate disclosure or promoting too much equality.

Explanation of the rationale for specific questions and physical examination. Explaining your rationale for asking specific questions or doing parts of physical examination which may not seem logical to the patient is a similar skill to sharing your thoughts. It is another example of reducing uncertainty for the patient and again promotes a collaborative relationship. **Teach opportunistically** and use **role play** for **rehearsing** exact phrases to try out their effectiveness and acceptability. You can also ask learners **to sink themselves into the role of the patient** and ask them what they might think or feel if the doctor asks:

'Do your ankles swell?' (the patient presents with palpitations)
'How many pillows do you sleep with at night?' (the patient presents with shortness of breath)

or wants to examine parts of the body apparently unrelated to their complaints, for example examining the spleen of a patient who may have glandular fever or the neck of a patient who has a history of transient ischaemic attacks.

Explanation and planning

Problems that learners commonly experience in this part of the consultation are:

- omitting to discover the patient's ideas, thoughts and feelings, concerns and expectations earlier in the consultation
- forgetting to discover what the patient already knows
- giving too much information at once and using inappropriate language
- giving information and explanations or suggesting a management plan without checking whether the patient understands or agrees with it
- not involving patients collaboratively in shared decision making.

In our view, the explanation and planning part of the consultation is one of the most challenging sections to teach. New research evidence has become available which is often unfamiliar to learners and facilitators. In addition, this part of the interview is least likely to have been taught at undergraduate level. Yet if doctors get this part wrong, all their skill at gathering information and clinical reasoning may be for naught. For these reasons we suggest that course directors at all levels set time aside, at appropriate points in the course, specifically for exploring this section.

A number of useful strategies help learners focus and work constructively on explanation and planning:

- becoming familiar with the research evidence
- working out the objectives for this part of the consultation (see our companion volume, Chapter 5)
- working with set scenarios in which the focus of the interview is clearly on explanation and planning, for example a patient requesting hormone replacement therapy, preparing a patient for a test to detect cancer of the prostate or presenting and discussing the results of investigations
- working with well-trained, simulated patients portraying cases which allow learners to explore explanation and planning.

PROVIDING THE CORRECT AMOUNT AND TYPE OF INFORMATION

Chunking and checking. It is common to see learners delivering long monologues to patients when they are giving information. Often there is much useful content, but after even as short a time as 30 seconds the patient can look glazed and appear to be losing the thread of the doctor's comments. Facilitate the group to **describe** this accurately when looking at either a role play or a video and **link** the behaviour with the effect. **Role play** different ways of chunking the information into shorter pieces and then checking that the patient understands and agrees with the information or explanation given so far. Present **research evidence** that not all patients wish to receive the same amount of information.

Assessing the patient's starting point. Most learners have been in the position of giving information or instructions without finding out first what the patient already thinks and knows or has tried for himself. **Explain** that finding out the patient's starting point can reduce conflict in the consultation and save time. If this can be explored experientially from the learner's agenda and demonstrated in a consultation, so much the better. **Role play** the group's suggestions and the patient's possible response:

'You asked me what high blood pressure is. Before I start, I'd like to ask what you know already about it.'
could produce a number of responses:
'Well doctor, my mother had high blood pressure and she took pills for it, but I never understood what they were supposed to do ...'
'My husband is a professor of biochemistry and has tried to explain it to me, so I've got some idea about it ... but ...'

ACHIEVING A SHARED UNDERSTANDING AND INCORPORATING THE PATIENT'S PERSPECTIVE

Relating explanations to the patient's ideas, concerns and expectations. **Consider as a group** one of Tuckett *et al.'s* (1985) main research conclusions that exploration of the patient's beliefs and ideas elicited earlier in the interview needs to be incorporated into the doctor's explanation in order to increase the patient's understanding and commitment. **Quote the research** of Korsch *et al.* (1968) and Eisenthal and Lazare (1976) who found that discovering patients' expectations led to increased patient satisfaction and the feeling of being helped, whether or not the expectations were met. Rehearse ways of linking patients' ideas, concerns and expectations discovered earlier in the consultation with giving information using **role play**.

Eliciting the patient's reactions and feelings. Once the explanation has been presented and the management plan discussed, prompt learners to discover how the patient has received or reacted to them. **Discuss the principle of effective communication** and how it is dependent on a two-way interaction; the doctor must check how the message has been received. This is particularly important whether breaking bad news to patients or simply discussing a prescription. Again, use **role play** to **rehearse** the phrases which learners suggest might be helpful to the patient in eliciting reactions to information given and plans under consideration.

PLANNING: SHARED DECISION MAKING

Involving the patient by making suggestions and offering choices. **Explore the advantages** of using these two skills with patients; for example, explore how making suggestions rather than giving directives and encouraging patients to make choices to the level that they wish may be helpful to both patient and doctor. **Quote the research evidence** from Fallowfield *et al.* (1990) that women with breast cancer who were seen by a specialist who favoured giving a choice to patients about their treatment suffered less depression and anxiety (even when technical considerations prevented a real choice) than women who were seen by surgeons who favoured either mastectomy or lumpectomy. **Brainstorm phrases** for making suggestions and offering choices which the learner can try in order to involve the patient:

'I'd like to make a suggestion here ...'
'What about trying ... What do you think?'
'Let's look at all the possibilities ...'
'I'd like to know which of these plans suits you best ...'
'Where would you like to go next ...'
'Tell me which of these options you'd like to try first ...'
'What do you favour here ...'

Negotiating a mutually acceptable plan and checking it with the patient. Ask the group to **work in pairs** and **think of scenarios** when the patient has not adhered to a plan (have some prepared yourself), and discuss the reasons for failure. **Refer to the research** of Coambs *et al.* (1995) and Meichenbaum and Turk (1987) which identifies factors contributing to adherence. **Link** the importance of summarizing and checking during the gathering-information stage of the consultation with their usefulness throughout the explanation and planning phase. Include their value in pulling together all the threads of an interactive process. **Identify and rehearse all the skills** which contribute to shared decision making between doctors and patients and reinforce those skills by referring to the appropriate sections of the *Calgary–Cambridge observation guide.*

Explanation and planning is a complicated process for both the patient and the doctor. Encourage learners to refer to the guide frequently and to ask themselves the following questions throughout this part of the interview in order to be sure they are covering both their own and the patient's perspective. Listing these questions for learners at the end of a teaching session on explanation and planning provides a **useful summary**:

- have I put myself in a position to give information?
- do I understand both my own and the patient's frames of reference?
- do I know what information I want to give?
- how can I phrase it in a way the patient can understand?
- does it relate to the patient's framework?
- how can I make sure that I am giving the information that the patient needs and wants?
- how can I check?

Ending the interview

Problems for doctors in this section of the interview often concern:

- time management
- late-arising complaints or problems
- failing to reiterate next steps and allow time for questions.

A satisfactory conclusion is dependent on effective consulting in the rest of the consultation. One way of exploring these links is to use **paired listening, brainstorming, a round** or **discussion** of the following two questions:

1 What helps the end of a consultation to proceed satisfactorily?
2 What hinders or gets in the way of an effective end to a consultation?

CONTRACTING, SAFETY NETTING AND FINAL CHECKING

Identifying next steps and individual responsibilities for both patient and doctor can be explored through **brainstorming, discussion in pairs** or **larger groups** and **flip charting** what the doctor and patient wish to achieve at this point in the consultation. Safety netting in the final steps of the consultation is crucial: **discuss** or **brainstorm** with the group the advantages to doctor and patient and follow with the disadvantages of failure to establish contingency plans. Ask the group to **describe scenarios** when safety netting was unexpectedly useful and the converse. **Role play** with a simulated patient the phrases a doctor might use in safety netting and check out their acceptability.

Communication issues

In our companion book, we include a chapter on specific communication issues in medicine and use breaking bad news, interviewing mentally ill patients and exploring cultural issues as examples. Most books on communication in medicine spend little time on core communication skills before moving quickly on to describing how to perform the medical interview in various specific circumstances. We have taken the opposite approach in our two books. If core skills are mastered first then more complex issues become very much easier to tackle. Below are some ways to explore three communication issues from the point of view of identifying the *core skills* and the *issue-specific skills* and seeing how these fit into the overall framework of the consultation. Exploring specific issues provides an ideal opportunity to integrate learning about skills and attitudes. For other communication issues, see Chapter 9 of this book or Chapter 7 of *Skills for Communicating with Patients*.

BREAKING BAD NEWS

The core skills of explanation and planning provide almost all the skills necessary to tackle the difficult task of breaking bad news.

Role play using simulated patients or group members is useful here. Try **prepared role plays** of breaking bad news about serious illness, for example cancer, death from a heart attack of a close relative or an inevitable miscarriage. If the learners are role playing, allow time for preparing the 'patient' as well as the 'doctor'. Using an observer and **working in trios** helps to encourage learners to take the exercise seriously; performing this type of role in front of the whole group can be threatening and needs a safe and supportive environment. Use **agenda-led, outcome-based analysis**, including **feedback from the patient. Refer to the explanation and planning part of the guide. Discuss** those skills which worked well and those which did not and re-rehearse. **Summarize** and work out with the group which skills are core skills and which are issue specific. The latter might include:

- giving a warning shot first
- knowing when to stop because the patient does not wish to or cannot hear more ('shut down')
- interviewing more than one person at a time
- co-partnership and advocacy
- giving hope tempered with realism
- the learner not coping appropriately with her own distress.

Flip chart other circumstances of breaking bad news which the learner may think are less serious but the patient may perceive otherwise: for example, giving the diagnosis of hypothyroidism, an abnormal cervical smear result or that the patient needs treatment for, say, hypertension. Rehearse using **role play or simulated patients**.

Work out a framework for breaking bad news (see Chapter 7 of our companion book) and **distribute a handout** later to reinforce learning. **Discuss the research evidence** for doctors' deficiencies in giving bad or difficult news (Finlay and Dallimore 1991, and numerous articles in the medical and lay press).

INTERVIEWING THE PSYCHOTIC AND DEPRESSED PATIENT

Many learners lack confidence in interviewing mentally ill patients. **Pairs exercises** and **discussion** about difficulties and fears of consulting patients who are psychotic or deeply depressed can uncover a number of personal and professional blocks to empathizing and communicating well with these patients. Try a **patient-centred exercise** of how it might feel to have disordered thinking or to be suicidal; link it with what it might feel like going to see the doctor and what the needs of the doctor might be. Give learners enough time to sink themselves into the role, perhaps getting them to think of a patient they have known or even when they themselves were depressed, and then speak to a partner as if they were the patient. **Flip chart** the feelings and the needs that come up from each pair. Allow enough time for safe **discussion**. Encourage the group to summarize the core skills and link them to the guides. Core skills here might be: listening, asking directed questions, gauging the patient's emotional state, demonstrating empathy, picking up cues, encouraging the patient to 'open up' and other skills needed to build up the relationship with the patient, for example proceeding at the patient's pace and providing clear explanations.

Work out with the group which issue-specific skills they find difficult but which are essential to use, for example uncovering hidden depression, assessing suicidal risk, assessing disordered thinking or beliefs. **Role play phrases** which the group find helpful. The use of **simulated patients** with psychotic illness is very helpful in this context, assuming that they are well trained.

Cultural Issues

The core communication skills which are essential for doctors to use when interviewing a patient from a culture other than their own – or when trying to understand the health-related beliefs of patients from their own culture – are those which discover the patient's framework in terms of beliefs, ideas, concerns and expectations of the medical encounter. Ask learners to give **examples of problems** which they have encountered in this area and relate them to the disease–illness model (McWhinney 1989). Use **patient-centred exercises** to help learners with empathy in relation to their ethnic patients by asking them to sink themselves into the following roles and explore the issues through **role play** (Eleftheriadou 1996):

- a recently arrived immigrant with little language facility who has to attend an emergency centre with a possible fracture
- a Muslim couple who are unexpectedly infertile
- a Hindu woman who wishes to see a female doctor but there is none available
- a patient who needs an interpreter
- a patient from the learner's own culture who has health beliefs that differ from the learner's.

Simulated patients who can **role play** ethnic patients convincingly are helpful, as are real patients or learners from ethnic backgrounds who can tell their stories of medical encounters. Gill and Adshead (1996) have developed a module for teaching cultural aspects of health which includes **interviewing patients at home**. Evaluation of this module has shown that learners have increased awareness of the communication difficulties which may occur in interviews where cultural issues arise. Littlewood and Lipsedge (1993) provide an excellent *text for discussion* of commonly occurring mismatches between doctors' and patients' belief systems, particularly in relation to cultural issues and the effects of immigration.

Part 3

Constructing a communication skills curriculum

8

Designing the programme

Introduction

We now move away from the facilitation of individual sessions and look at the communication skills curriculum as a whole. We consider how to convert the approaches to teaching and learning described in this book so far into communication skills programmes that will produce effective and long-lasting change in learners' communication skills. How can we translate our understanding of what to teach and which methods of learning to employ into a well-designed curriculum? How do we organize a coherent programme that ensures systematic and ongoing skill development in both training and clinical practice? How can we construct a comprehensive, well-organized curriculum when problem-based, experiential learning is so opportunistic and non-sequential?

In this chapter we explore how to construct a communication skills curriculum in practice by:

- providing a conceptual framework for systematic communication training
- identifying issues and questions common to the design of all communication curricula
- offering strategies and principles that help address these issues.

Throughout this book and its companion volume we have stressed the common ground in communication teaching and learning throughout medical education – the underlying principles and concepts, theory and research evidence, core skills, teaching methods and facilitation techniques. In this chapter we demonstrate that issues of curriculum design also remain constant across all levels of medical education, in all specialties and in a wide variety of countries. That is not to say that one single standardized communication course will suit all circumstances. We serve a varied array of professionals and patients communicating in many contexts. Curricula need to be tailored to the particular needs of individual patients and learners. Yet, once again there is common ground: the need to consider where particular learners at any level are starting from and to build our communication programmes from that base.

A conceptual framework for systematic communication training

Carroll and Monroe (1979), Kurtz (1989), Simpson *et al.* (1991) and Seely *et al.* (1995) have all highlighted the importance of structured communication skills programmes which include an explicit statement of the skills to be learned and evaluated and in which specific skills are identified and practised. A systematic approach to the development of communication programmes is necessary.

As a first step in this process we have found it helpful to devise a simple framework for systematic communication training which pulls together many of the central elements of communication teaching and learning covered in this book so far (Box 8.1). This framework provides a template to help us think through how to organize the curriculum and decide on approaches to assessment. Together with the *Calgary–Cambridge observation guide*, the framework forms the common foundation for all the communication curricula that we have developed on both sides of the Atlantic, whether for medical students, residents or practising physicians.

We have already explored the first three components of this framework in Part 1 of this book. The final component requires further elaboration. We have found it helpful in planning and programme development to keep in mind four focuses of learning and assessment (Miller 1990): knowledge, competence, performance and results. All are important in physician–patient communication. Knowledge and competence can and must be taught and evaluated in medical school and then reviewed, refined, deepened and added to in helical fashion during residency and CME. Performance and results, however, can only be tackled during residency and CME where we can see what doctors actually choose to do with patients and what the outcomes of these choices are. We must therefore extend communication training into upper levels of medical education and coordinate that training with undergraduate communication programmes.

Issues in curriculum design and implementation

Over the last two decades there has been considerable and increasing pressure from professional medical bodies to improve the training and evaluation of doctors in communication at both national (General Medical Council 1978, 1993; Association of American Medical Colleges 1984; American Board of Pediatrics 1987; Workshop Planning Committee 1992; Cowan and Laidlaw 1993; Barkun 1995; Royal College of Physicians 1997) and international levels (World Federation for Medical Education 1994). Many medical schools and institutions throughout the world have heeded this advice and have set up formal communication training courses as part of their educational programmes. Despite this welcome and substantial progress, a number of issues continue to challenge programme directors working to design and implement first-class communication programmes in medical education (Kurtz 1989; Whitehouse 1991; Novack *et al.* 1993). How do we:

- **develop the communication curriculum?**
  - ensure learners not only master an increasing range of skills but also retain and use them over time?

Box 8.1 A conceptual framework for systematic communication training

---

Underlying assumptions
- Communication is a basic clinical skill.
- Communication in medicine is a series of learned skills rather than a personality trait – anyone who wants to can learn them.
- Experience can be a poor teacher of communication skills.
- Certain specific learning methods are essential to obtain change:
  - observation
  - well-intentioned, detailed and descriptive feedback
  - rehearsal of skills.

Organizational schema for communication programmes (*Riccardi and Kurtz 1983*)
Goals of medical communication:
- Accuracy
- Efficiency
- Supportiveness

Tasks of the medical interview:
- Initiating the session
- Gathering information
- Building the relationship
- Explanation and planning
- Closing the session

Broad categories of skills:
- Content skills – what doctors do
- Process skills – how they do it
- Perceptual skills – what they are thinking and feeling

Principles that characterize effective communication (*Kurtz 1989*)
- Ensures an interaction rather than a direct transmission process
- Reduces unnecessary uncertainty
- Requires planning and thinking in terms of outcomes
- Demonstrates dynamism
- Follows the helical model

Focuses of learning and assessment (*Miller 1990*)
- Knowledge – do you know it?
- Competence – can you do it?
- Performance – do you (choose to) do it in practice?
- Results – what happens to the patients and to the doctors?

- select and organize the content of communication programmes (*decide on the core communication content, tailor and organize content in relation to particular learners' needs* and *ensure a balance between all components of the programme*)?
- select appropriate teaching methods for each component of the programme?
- integrate communication with other clinical skills and the rest of the learners' curriculum?
- **assess learners' communication skills effectively and efficiently?**
  - develop formative assessment as part of the communication programme?
  - develop summative, certifying assessment of communication skills?
- **promote the further development and acceptance of communication curricula within medical education?**
  - find adequate time and resources for communication training in an already over-burdened medical curriculum?
  - coordinate communication curricula at all levels of medical education?
  - ensure the status of communication training as a bona fide clinical skill across all specialties?
- **enhance facilitator skills?**
  - enhance facilitators' own communication skills with patients?
  - increase their knowledge base about communication skills, theory and research?
  - enhance their communication teaching and facilitation skills?
  - maximize the status and reward of undertaking such teaching?

Chapters 8 and 9 consider each of these issues in turn. This chapter addresses two issues, curriculum development and assessment of learners' communication skills. Chapter 9 examines ways to promote the further development of communication curricula in medical education and enhance facilitator training.

SECTION 1: DEVELOPING THE COMMUNICATION CURRICULUM

How do we ensure that learners not only master an increasing range of skills but also retain and use them over time?

We have already demonstrated that doctor–patient communication is a complicated process with an extensive curriculum of communication skills for doctors to master and put into practice in the real world. How do we design communication curricula that enable learners to assimilate these skills? How do we ensure that learners gradually increase and extend their repertoire of communication skills? And how can we enable them to retain these skills over time so that they actually use them to effect in their future practice?

Three overriding principles of programme design help us to address these questions and to guide our overall planning of communication skills programmes.

A curriculum rather than a course

Many of the problems of current communication skills teaching stem from the common tendency to structure communication training into a single, self-contained course, frequently offered near the beginning of the overall teaching programme and separated from the teaching of other clinical skills. Commonly, this course concludes with a single assessment of what students have learned in isolation from the rest of the medical curriculum. Yet to achieve a significant and lasting impact on learners' communication skills, we need more than a one-off course. Learners' communication needs change and develop as they progress through training and increase their levels of intellectual and clinical sophistication. Our teaching interventions therefore need to be appropriately timed: it is not possible to address all our learners' communication requirements at any single point in their educational programme. For instance, in medical school, the emphasis of the communication programme moves gradually from beginning the interview and building the relationship to information gathering and then on to explanation and planning. Because learners' communication requirements cannot be addressed at any single point, programme directors must plan a curriculum with multiple components that recur at intervals within each level and throughout learners' education as a whole.

A helical rather than linear curriculum

Just as a one-off module is not enough, neither are sequential modules that do not allow the learner to revisit areas previously covered.

There is clear evidence that communication skills once learned are easily forgotten. Engler *et al.* (1981) demonstrated that students' skills improved significantly following interviewing skills training in their first year of medical school but declined just as significantly by the second year without further reinforcement. Craig (1992) found that students who had attended an optional interviewing course in their first year improved significantly over a control group but over the next three years this improvement began to evaporate and eventually all gains over the control group were lost. However, Kauss *et al.* (1980) showed that residents from medical schools which provided more comprehensive interpersonal skills courses (for instance, using videotape in more than just an introductory course) were significantly better at eliciting and dealing with emotional material than residents from other schools. Residents from schools with more limited interpersonal skills courses actually fared worse than those with no interpersonal training at all. Kraan *et al.* (1990) have since demonstrated that sustained benefits can be achieved using a comprehensive and continuous format of interviewing skills training over a four-year period.

These studies conclude that communication skills learning must be reiterated throughout learners' clinical training. Two features of medical education may account for this. First, any initial emphasis on communication skills appears to be swamped as students struggle to come to grips with medical problem solving; preoccupation with the disease process needs to be repeatedly counterbalanced by communication skills training or gains in learners' communication skills are lost (Kraan *et al.* 1990). Second, as many experienced clinicians have received little education themselves in communication skills and may even denigrate the importance of interview skills training, poor role modelling from clinicians in practice may counter the effect of formal communication training programmes.

There are, however, even more fundamental reasons for making sure students revisit their previous communication skills learning as the course proceeds. A basic educational principle indicates that communication skills learning needs to take a helical rather than linear path

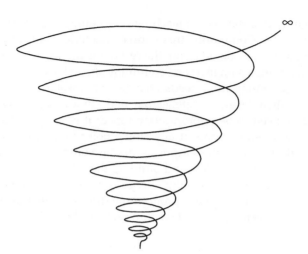

∞

Fig 8.1 Dance (1967) model of communication

(Fig. 8.1) (Dance 1967; Riccardi and Kurtz 1983; Kurtz 1989). Earlier in this book we introduced the helix as an important theoretical principle of communication. Here we apply the helical model to learning and curriculum design. Helical learning is the foundation of all our planning and implementation strategies. It suggests that learners need to do more than just complete one module of the communication course and then move on to another isolated component. Learning communication skills is not achieved after a single exposure. Repetition and review of previous learning are required for maximum skill development. The well-planned curriculum provides opportunities for learners to review, refine and build on existing skills while at the same time adding in new skills and increasing complexity so that the learner comes around the spiral of learning at a slightly higher level each time.

Why is this reiteration so necessary? Because people learn in helical rather than linear fashion. Think about a time when you learned a new skill like playing golf, the piano or speaking a new language. To learn it well you needed to do more than go to a series of lessons, each on a different topic, one following the other with no reiteration or review on the assumption that once something had been presented, it was done. The linear model does not match the way people learn. We require introduction, reiteration and review, opportunities to try things out, to be challenged with increasing complexity, to succeed and to fail safely, to drill, to build on existing skills, even to relearn.

Planning curricula around the helical model of built-in reiteration, gradual refinement and increasing sophistication helps to ensure that learners not only master skills but retain and use them over time. Without ongoing and helical communication programmes running throughout the learner's course as a whole, students will forget or fail to master communication skills to a professional level. A helical curriculum also helps to overcome one of the key challenges of communication skills teaching, namely how to plan a programme in the context of opportunistic experiential learning where it is not entirely possible to predetermine what skills will be covered. A helical programme allows for those areas that by chance have not been addressed in a particular session to surface later. Facilitators can take comfort that when opportunities pass by, they are not lost forever. In Appendix 1, we provide examples of undergraduate and residency curricula built on the helical model.

Integrated, not separated, from the rest of the medical curriculum

The third principle of programme design is to ensure that communication skills are actively integrated both with learners' training in other clinical skills and with other parts of the medical curriculum. Self-contained communication courses with their major focus on communication and with facilitators who understand communication teaching and learning are essential. Without them, communication tends to receive inadequate attention. But integrating communication back into the larger medical curriculum is also important so that communication is not perceived as a separate entity divorced from real medicine (Carroll and Monroe 1979; Engler *et al.* 1981; Kurtz 1989; van Dalen *et al.* 1989). Without integration, communication can look like an inessential frill rather than a basic clinical skill relevant to all encounters with patients. Furthermore, if we want communication to be seen as a bona fide subject applicable to all disciplines, then it must be taught not only in primary care or psychiatry but also in other specialty areas and with the active help of doctors from a wide range of disciplines. We discuss approaches to integration in greater detail later in this chapter.

How do we select and organize the content of our communication programmes?

Deciding on the core content of the programme

In Part 1 of this book, we presented our rationale for taking a skills-based approach to communication teaching and described the core skills that together constitute the communication curriculum. The *Calgary–Cambridge observation guide* summarizes these skills.

This core content of communication skills is the same across all three levels of medical education (undergraduate, residency and continuing medical education) and across many diverse medical contexts. This point can appear to be counterintuitive: many specialty groups that we have worked with have initially suggested that the communication skills required in their particular setting are unique. But in fact the core skills are truly neither context nor level specific. While different contexts may require a subtle shift in emphasis or adaptation of skills to suit the specific needs of doctors and patients in those particular circumstances, the underlying principles and core communication skills remain the same and form a common base for all communication curricula.

Tailoring and organizing the content in relation to learners' needs

When planning a communication curriculum, the focus and sequence of learning are often more difficult to come to grips with than the individual skills. Although the core skills of communication programmes remain constant throughout all three levels of medical education, there is still considerable variation in:

- the overall communication needs of each group of learners
- the specific content required at their particular stage of learning
- the sequence in which this content is best presented.

The design of each communication curriculum must therefore be carefully adapted to the needs of your particular learners.

WHO ARE YOUR LEARNERS?

When planning a curriculum, first take account of who your learners are:

- at what stage in their career are they?
- what are their specific communication needs?
- what previous experience of communication skills teaching have they had?
- how uniform are their needs?

The level of medical education – undergraduate, residency or CME – is of particular importance. The communication needs of an undergraduate medical student, a resident and an established practitioner in the same specialty differ widely. Yet unlike many other fields in medicine, their communication needs are not purely determined by their experience – sometimes it is the most experienced practitioner who has the most basic needs.

UNDERGRADUATE MEDICAL EDUCATION

Overall learning needs

Because medical students begin with fewer preconceived ideas about doctor–patient communication than residents or practising physicians, determining the focus and sequence of the undergraduate communication curriculum is a relatively straightforward task. The following two areas need to be considered:

1 the agenda of the programme director and facilitators
   - core skills of the medical interview
   - selected issues
2 the agenda and problems of the participants themselves.

The agenda of the programme director and facilitators
Medical students have a reasonable base in communication from their outside world of non-medical experiences but limited understanding of either the content or process of medical interviewing. The curriculum therefore needs to lay strong foundations in all the tasks of the medical interview, starting from initiating and progressing through to closing the interview. Undergraduates can learn initiating the interview, gathering information and building the relationship in considerable depth. Explanation and planning cannot be covered in as much detail at this stage as in residency programmes but it *must* still be included in undergraduate education, as we discuss later in this chapter.

The undergraduate curriculum also has to explore communication issues and challenges such as ethics, culture, gender, dealing with emotions and death and dying. In medical schools which have modules outside the communication course dedicated to these issues, part of this responsibility may be met by coordinating efforts between courses.

The agenda and problems of the participants themselves
Medical students' motivation will be enhanced if the communication curriculum also addresses the problems that they themselves are experiencing or anticipate experiencing in their

contacts with patients and colleagues, both within the communication course and elsewhere. Facilitators need to identify learners' own communication needs and not just address a pre-planned agenda. However, certain skills and issues need to be introduced prior to learners experiencing difficulties in practice. For instance, explanation and planning, breaking bad news or confrontation are normally not entrusted to medical students and so direct experience of the difficulties posed by these tasks will not necessarily be obtained. Students need to gain protected experience of these skills and issues before they are faced with working them out with real patients.

Accomplishing this enormous agenda is a more daunting task than formulating it. A major decision for programme directors and facilitators is how much of the agenda to try to cover given that curriculum time is invariably restricted. There are compelling reasons for attempting to be as comprehensive as possible. If important areas of the interview such as explanation and planning or issues such as culture are left out of the undergraduate experience, students may not appreciate the importance of crucial skills and attitudes to effective medical practice. Furthermore, there is no guarantee in communication teaching at present that areas which receive little attention in medical school will in fact be taught later on in residency or CME. A final reason to strive for comprehensiveness in the undergraduate curriculum is that we are not just trying to maintain current expectations of communication competency but to advance the profession's standards of practice.

Organizing the content

In undergraduate medicine, a natural structure is imposed by learners' communication needs which helps to organize the curriculum. With limited initial understanding of either the content or process of medical interviewing, the medical student curriculum logically starts at the beginning of the consultation and can then gradually work through the medical interview. The curriculum can start with initiating the interview and building the relationship, progress to gathering information and the content of the medical interview (history of presenting complaint, past medical history, family history, social history, systems review, etc.), take in closing the interview and later on in the course tackle explanation and planning. Challenges posed for example by interviewing patients who are angry, depressed or in pain, can be included as the course progresses.

Despite this natural progression, the opportunistic nature of experiential learning still makes it difficult to ensure that particular skills are covered at any given point. Although we can decide the intended focus for each session in advance, we must still work from what actually happens in students' interviews and the learning agendas that surface. In addition, skills that are not reinforced are likely to atrophy once students leave the communication course; some of the experiences to which students are exposed outside the course can short-circuit even well-learned skills and attitudes. Planning is therefore not as straightforward as it may look. We can overcome these problems by structuring the curriculum to follow a helical rather than linear model, building repetition and reiteration into the programme even as we add new skills or greater complexity. In addition, we can provide frameworks like the one at the beginning of this chapter and the *Calgary–Cambridge observation guide* so that students and facilitators can see the bigger picture and identify the skills and issues on which they will be working over time.

Given the class sizes, a further organizational difficulty is how to generate not only the relevant content but also the sheer numbers of student–patient consultations needed for observation, analysis and practice in problem-based learning. Part of the solution lies in using a combination of real patients, simulated patients and role play along with video or audio recordings, as discussed in Chapter 4.

In Appendix 1, we provide an example of a helical problem-based communication curriculum in undergraduate medicine. This programme from the University of Calgary Faculty of Medicine spreads across the three-year medical school curriculum. The programme is primarily skills based and uses real patients, standardized patients and occasional student role play to provide the appropriate experiential material.

RESIDENCY AND CONTINUING MEDICAL EDUCATION

Overall learning needs

In residency and CME, determining the focus and sequence for communication curricula is more complicated. Here we see practitioners struggling with complex issues who have often had little previous formal instruction in the core skills of communication. Their training has frequently been gained only from their experience as doctors yet, as we have already seen, experience alone is often a poor teacher. So we have a potentially explosive mix of sophisticated and remedial education without any obvious sequence to learning.

Planning what to cover in a postgraduate communication curriculum is therefore a sensitive task that involves looking at three distinct areas:

1 remedial education: areas not covered that perhaps should have been many years ago or areas that have atrophied or been forgotten
2 the agendas of the programme director and facilitators: particular skills and issues that *you* consider worth exploring for doctors in a specific arena and at a particular stage of development
3 the agendas and problems of the doctors themselves: their stated needs that you might not consider without explicit discussion.

'Remedial' education

We do not mean this term in any pejorative sense – it is simply that many learners will have received little communication education in their undergraduate or postgraduate training and need time to explore and master the core skills of medical communication. This may well prove more difficult for established doctors than for medical students as often there is considerable unlearning to do and entrenched habits to overcome.

The agendas of the programme director and facilitators

From the programme director's perspective, substantial common ground often exists between the needs of both residents and experienced practitioners in any one specialty. Components to include in communication programmes for either group include:

• review and refinement of initiation, relationship building and gathering information: those who have been fortunate to have experienced the benefit of communication training need these areas reinforced and built upon in helical fashion
• explanation and planning: many programmes at undergraduate level will not have taught this vital subject in any detail. Even if undergraduate programmes do teach it, learners have

too little medical technical knowledge and experience prior to residency training to undertake comprehensive explanation and planning with real patients, much less to develop these skills in depth. Because these skills can only be fully explored during residency and CME, explanation and planning should be a prime focus of communication skills training at postgraduate level

- specific issues: these will vary from specialty to specialty and depend on learners' individual needs. Possibilities include breaking bad news, chronic illness, revealing hidden depression, ethics, prevention, addiction, third-party consultations with the patient's family or friends and communication between team members or between specialists and primary care doctors.

The agendas and problems of the doctors themselves
In contrast to the programme director's view, residents and more experienced practitioners often differ markedly in their expressed communication needs. For instance, early in their training, residents in family practice, removed from the apparent safety of the student's role and faced with complex decision making in practice, express particular difficulty with the focused interview, with uncertainty, with the unstructured nature of general practice and with dealing with patients rather than just diseases. They are uncomfortable with much of the subject matter of general practice and feel unsafe with both the content and process of their work. In contrast, established practitioners feel more comfortable with content but express difficulties with complex, long-standing patients, with heart-sink patients, with empathy and with the pressures they face from a busy and demanding system that does not allow them to perform at their best (Levinson *et al.* 1993). Time is often their utmost concern.

Similar differences between the expressed needs of residents and senior doctors are found in other specialties. Rheumatology residents struggle with obtaining histories quickly and accurately from anxious, newly referred patients and face the added difficulty of relative lack of knowledge. They may have problems in explaining the inconclusive nature of many of their investigations and have difficulties in knowing how to deal with chronic medical problems which lie outside their specialist area. They may be uncertain how to discuss evidence with patients, especially when the patients present complex data searched out on the Internet. In contrast, experienced rheumatologists may be battling against time pressures, having difficulty dealing with problems such as chronic back pain where no physical illness is apparent or coping with angry patients for whom medicine does not have an answer and where there is a possibility of medico-legal complaint.

Organizing the content
In residency and CME, organizing content is less straightforward than in undergraduate medicine. At first glance, taking into account the importance of a structured curriculum and the potential need for remedial education, it would again seem appropriate for the curriculum to start with simple skills and for the level of complexity to increase as the programme develops. Unfortunately, this does not take into account the perceived needs, concerns and sensibilities of the experienced doctor. Struggling with complex issues, practising doctors will not appreciate having to start with apparently lower level skills such as how to initiate a consultation, even if there are important skills here which they are unaware of that could help considerably in the accuracy, efficiency and supportiveness of their interviews: *'Of course I know how to begin an interview, I've already done 75 000!'*.

The problem here is that if we start at the bottom, from scratch, we are taking an approach that some experienced physicians will perceive as demeaning. Yet if we start from the seventh floor, we have not built any foundations. This is a difficult balance, exacerbated by the particular problems of teaching practising doctors. They have:

- further to fall
- more potential unlearning
- more ingrained habits

and are often more threatened by communication skills programmes. And the more experienced the doctor, the more difficult these problems may become. Experienced doctors who have practised medicine for many years may not be particularly keen to have an expert challenging what they have become comfortable in doing: *'I get by, why change? If you're saying I can improve, doesn't it imply that I haven't been doing it very well these last 20 years?'*.

So, as with all adult learning, it is best to take a problem-based approach which seems relevant and therefore acceptable to learners. We cannot start from the bottom and work up without creating defensiveness. Instead, start from where participants are and work both up and down. We need to start with problems participants face in their own practice of medicine yet make sure that we explore the lower levels of the communication skills ladder. This is not as difficult as it may seem – as we have said, even the most complex problems more often than not relate to core communication skills such as listening, question style, structuring, empathy, picking up cues and body language. Even with complicated issues, the answer to problems will usually lie in core communication skills that form the very nub of effective communication.

This means that communication programmes must take a problem-based approach in the first instance, tackling the participant's agenda initially, gently and opportunistically introducing work on specific skills and later introducing more planned work on sections of the consultation and specific issues in communication. Lacking the natural progression of undergraduate programmes, structuring and organizing learning over time becomes a more difficult problem for organizers, facilitators and learners. Concise frameworks for skills and the curriculum, such as the *Calgary–Cambridge observation guide*, become indispensable.

In Appendix 1, we present an example of a residency programme where this problem-based approach to learning has been adopted.

Ensuring a balance between all relevant aspects of the communication curriculum

The issue of balance in planning communication programmes arises primarily in two areas:

1 how to combine the teaching of communication issues, attitudes and skills
2 where and how to teach explanation and planning.

BALANCING COMMUNICATION SKILLS, ATTITUDES AND ISSUES

As discussed in Chapter 3, the well-rounded communication curriculum deals with three overlapping areas:

1 skills (content, process and perceptual)

2 attitudes

3 issues.

How do we ensure an appropriate balance between these three vital components? This book deliberately focuses on a skills-based approach to communication teaching and learning. Here, we explore how to address attitudes and issues within this skills-based environment.

Attitudinal work

Attitudes are important and need careful attention in communication programmes. How can we combine the teaching of complementary skills and attitudes within a skills-based curriculum? Here are two possible approaches that can be taken:

1 *Discussion during skills-based teaching sessions.* The first approach is to enable attitudes to surface during skills-based teaching sessions. As learners give and receive feedback about their communication skills, ample opportunities arise to encourage discussion of underlying attitudes and assumptions that influence how learners communicate with patients. Capitalize on these opportunities by encouraging learners to openly discuss attitudes which appear to be either helpful or problematical. Attitudes towards a patient-centred approach, dealing with difficult emotions, sharing information with patients, specific groups of patients such as those with HIV or alcoholism, patients making inappropriate demands, 'trivial illness', and the relationship between what learners are discovering about communication and their perception of what is possible in the real world can all be aired.

Questions can be raised about learners' perceptions of their own attitudes or assumptions and the effect these often subconscious variables have on what the learner and the patient are doing or saying. One approach for opening fruitful consideration of attitudes is to ask the learner *'What outcome do you want to achieve?'* at the specific point in the consultation where difficulties appear to be emerging. Comparing different possible outcomes will highlight attitudinal variations in a non-judgemental way, e.g. *'to get the patient out of the room and never see him again'* or *'to look at the long term and build a relationship'*. Once learners identify outcomes, it becomes easier to discuss attitudes openly and explore the corresponding actions and skills that will lead to different end results. This kind of explicit discussion can lead to significant changes in both attitudes and skills.

2 *Devoting specific sessions to the discussion of attitudes.* A second approach is to hold separate sessions within the communication unit which focus specifically on attitudes. Alternative forums for these discussions include Balint-like awareness groups or the well physician programmes that some medical schools have instituted. In addition to those listed above, topics include:

- difficulties with challenging or confronting patients
- needing to be liked
- wishing to be in control
- feeling helpless
- our own emotions
- our own and our patients' sexuality.

Attitudes and problems can be discussed in relation to our own underlying personalities and upbringing, previous life experiences and personal prejudices. These approaches can all lead to fruitful reflection about blocks or restrictive attitudes.

However, we must ensure that such sessions move beyond discussion of attitudes to work on appropriately linked skills. There is little point in raising awareness about attitudes or even describing more useful approaches without also offering the skills for resolving problems and for putting alternatives into practice. Why change attitudes towards, say, addicted patients without providing learners with the opportunity to develop the skills to be both empathic and firm? As we stated in Chapter 3, although attitude work is important in raising awareness, it is impotent in effecting useful change in learners' behaviour without the addition of skills training. A participant in one of our workshops made this point beautifully. He described how excited he had become about patient-centred medicine as a result of a two-year masters course which discussed patient-centred medicine in detail and the research surrounding it. He became committed to the idea of making his practice more patient centred, yet despite his best intentions and his certainty that it would serve both him and his patients better, nothing changed. During a subsequent three-day seminar working on the skills described in the *Calgary–Cambridge observation guide*, he realized that what he had been missing was work on the *skills* needed to implement the patient-centred approach.

Communication issues

Communication skills programmes also need to provide learners with exposure to specific communication issues and challenges, for instance:

- ethics
- culture
- gender
- age
- special needs patients
- difficult situations
- chronic/acute care
- death and dying
- health promotion and prevention.

How can we address these specific issues in skills-based programmes?

Introducing issues into relevant components of a skills-based communication curriculum

As we described in Chapter 3, this book takes a predominantly skills- rather than issues-based approach to communication skills teaching and learning. Although specific issues may call for special adaptations and even additional skills, the core skills of the *Calgary–Cambridge observation guide* are still very much the primary resource needed for effective management of all these communication issues and challenges. We therefore prefer to base our programmes on the exploration of core skills, using specific communication issues to discover first how these core skills can be employed in particular circumstances and then what issue-specific skills need to be superimposed upon them. The strategy which we use most frequently here is the development of simulated patient cases that present learners with specific issues or challenges relevant to appropriate sections of the interview. For example, one of our standardized patient cases is an Asian woman seen in the emergency room who is having trouble speaking; her problem is not difficulty with English, as the clinician who saw her in real life thought, but a neurological problem that has interfered with her speech. A second is a married Latino woman of childbearing age who may need to consider a hysterectomy. These simulations provide an opportunity to explore culture and gender issues as part of our teaching on information-gathering skills. Similarly, the issues of breaking bad news or motivation of change can be dealt with as part of our teaching on the skills of explanation and planning. We can also work on issues in a less planned way with material that arises serendipitously in interviews with real patients.

Building the communication curriculum around issues
An alternative approach is to construct the curriculum entirely around issues, with each session (or series of sessions) focusing on a specific issue. Some residency and CME programmes have used this approach as a motivating device to help establish communication programmes. For example, a residency programme for general and orthopaedic surgeons discovered through a needs assessment that residents wanted to learn strategies to approach the issues of informed consent and breaking bad news to patients. Communication training for these residents therefore began with those two issues and the skills required to deal with them (Descouteaux 1996).

Collaborating with other issues-orientated courses
Another strategy for dealing with communication issues is to collaborate with colleagues who direct specific issues-orientated courses or seminars. We can, for instance, collaborate on developing joint objective standardized clinical evaluation (OSCE) stations for certifying evaluations that serve both communication and ethics programmes.

ENSURING ADEQUATE EMPHASIS ON EXPLANATION AND PLANNING

At all levels of training, communication programmes have tended to concentrate on gathering information and relationship-building skills and underplay the importance of explanation and planning. Despite its crucial importance to outcomes of care, this area of communication training remains largely underdeveloped (Carroll and Monroe 1979; Kahn *et al*. 1979; Simpson *et al*. 1991). The tendency to emphasize information gathering and relationship building is understandable. Much of the earlier research focused on these skills rather than those of explanation and planning. Furthermore, information-gathering skills are easier and safer to teach to undergraduates (where most communication training has been undertaken until recently) than the skills of explanation and planning.

Two developments have improved our ability to teach explanation and planning. The first is the explosion in the last decade of research and theoretical literature concerning this section of the medical interview. This has provided us with a far stronger basis for developing teaching programmes in this area (see Maguire *et al*. 1986b; Ley 1988; Kaplan *et al*. 1989; Roter and Hall 1992 and numerous references in Chapter 5 of our companion volume). The second development has been the increasingly widespread use of simulated patients. While medical students are provided with innumerable situations in which to take histories from patients (although, unfortunately, often without the benefit of observation and feedback), the same is certainly not true of giving information. Students do not generally know enough to be trusted to give information to real patients or answer their questions about their care and neither physicians nor patients wish students to experiment and make mistakes. This encourages undergraduates to develop the mistaken notion that communication with patients is primarily about history taking or detective work. The use of standardized patients helps correct this imbalance by providing opportunities for practice and rehearsal of explanation and planning skills that are safe for patients and students, even if learners have knowledge gaps or give incorrect information. This strategy is useful with all levels of learners.

Undergraduate education can and should establish a strong foundation in the area of explanation and planning. However, because undergraduates do not normally have a formal role in management or responsibility for patient care, reinforcement and full development of these skills must take place during residency and CME.

ADAPTING THE CALGARY–CAMBRIDGE OBSERVATION GUIDE FOR DIFFERENT LEVELS

The *Calgary–Cambridge observation guide* provides another useful tool for achieving an appropriate balance in communication programmes. The guide identifies the communication skills for each task of the interview and, in effect, summarizes the available research. With this concise and visible representation, it becomes relatively easy to check any programme in the planning stages to ensure that all areas of the interview are emphasized appropriately.

We have found it necessary to vary the use of the *Calgary–Cambridge observation guide* to reflect the differences, outlined above, in content, organization and balance of communication curricula in the three levels of medical education. Although the guide is equally useful for teaching in undergraduate, residency and CME, the different contexts and the particular thrust of the teaching in these three settings need to be mirrored in the format of the guide and the intensity of focus on particular skills.

Undergraduate medical education

The *Calgary–Cambridge observation guide* was originally developed as two independent guides (Guide One: Interviewing the Patient and Guide Two: Explanation and Planning) used separately within the undergraduate communication curriculum at the University of Calgary. The two-guide format enables undergraduates to:

- work with a manageable number of skills at any given time
- focus on history taking and relationship building for the first part of the programme
- add the skills of explanation and planning as the course progresses.

We still recommend using these two separate guides in undergraduate medical education and include these versions in Appendix 2 of this book.

Guide One is specifically geared to consultations which focus primarily on information gathering and is thus ideally suited to the initial stages of undergraduate medical education. We include the guide in core document materials which students receive before classes begin. Covering all five tasks of the interview but only a limited number of items on explanation and planning and a composite of items on closing the session, Guide One is the basis of the communication programme over the first year.

The communication programme spreads across the three-year medical school curriculum and we introduce Guide Two part way through the second year when we begin to shift the focus from gathering information to explanation and planning. This guide focuses directly on explanation and planning and expands closing the session. The second guide can be used alone but is often used in conjunction with the first guide for two reasons: firstly, many of the problems doctors encounter with explanation and planning have their origins in what occurred during initiation, information gathering and relationship building; and secondly, by the time we get to the later phases of our programme it is clear that students need reiteration, review and deepening of the communication skills that they learned in the earlier phases of the programme.

Residency and continuing medical education

In residency and CME, we use either the two separate guides described above or the combined version presented in Chapter 2.

In some circumstances, such as out-patient work in specialist medicine, interviews tend to divide into one of two basic types. In the first, the primary focus is on history taking and evaluation of problems. This would include not only the evaluation of a new problem but also the follow-up of patients with acute or chronic problems to assess progress or the outcome of treatment. Using Guide One by itself is particularly appropriate here, even though some explanation and planning will feature, for instance in describing preliminary opinions, preparation for tests or explaining next steps.

Guide Two is especially useful in the second situation where explanation and planning is the main purpose of the interview, such as the patient's follow-up visit to discuss the results of tests. However, even in this type of consultation, all the original tasks in Guide One still pertain and many of the skills listed in Guide One are still applicable. In particular, the tasks of initiation, building the relationship and facilitating the patient's involvement are crucial to effective explanation and planning.

For other circumstances, for instance in teaching family medicine residents, dermatologists, rheumatologists, genito-urinary specialists and now even cardiologists (where the ready availability of echocardiograms within out-patient practice can enable the doctor to provide immediate answers at the initial meeting), we have produced the combined version of the guides that appears in Chapter 2. Many of these consultations progress from information gathering to definitive explanation and planning in one meeting. This combined version covers all the skills of the medical interview together.

How do we select appropriate methods for each component of the communication programme?

The choice of teaching and learning methods significantly influences the outcomes which a communication programme or any of its individual sessions achieves. The programme director needs to incorporate an appropriate combination of methods, depending on their availability, cost, suitability to a specific session and the availability of curriculum time. This important area is examined in depth in Chapter 4.

How do we integrate communication with other clinical skills and the rest of the curriculum?

Earlier in this chapter we advocated integrating the communication skills programme with learners' training in other clinical skills and with other components of the medical curriculum.

Communication needs to be an integral part of the medical curriculum, not a separate entity divorced from 'real medicine' and taught only in separate self-contained courses. It is vital to integrate all four areas of medical practice which together determine overall clinical competence:

1 knowledge
2 communication skills
3 problem solving
4 physical examination.

Learners will benefit if this is a two-way process, that is, if the communication programme considers how to incorporate and address other relevant clinical skills *and* if other components of the overall curriculum address communication whenever it is relevant. Explicit coordination and discussion between individuals working with the various components is necessary to accomplish this.

Strategies which facilitate the integration of communication and other clinical skills include:

- dividing the communication curriculum into segments which can be offered at intervals across the overall medical curriculum rather than all at one time
- intentionally integrating communication with other clinical skills and with learners' expanding knowledge
- devising a summary of skills – such as the *Calgary–Cambridge observation guide* – which concisely conveys to other course directors or facilitators the core content of the communication curriculum so that they can build on or use it where applicable in their courses
- bringing other coursework into the communication programme, for example through the use of simulated patients who portray ethics problems or problems related to issues of culture or gender or specific medical problems that students are studying simultaneous to the communication course
- designing learning exercises and evaluations as close as possible to actual clinical settings wherein students must integrate communication with other skills in order to solve patient problems.

Combining content, process and perceptual issues

In medical education it is all too easy to assume that the learning has been achieved once the issues of knowledge, physical examination and problem solving have been discussed. Yet so often this omits an area of medical practice essential to completing the task effectively: communicating with the patient. Imagine a tutorial for surgical residents concerning the diagnosis and management of breast cancer. Certainly the discussion would be wanting if it did not include an analysis of disease and pathology, of physical examination technique and investigation and treatment. However, is it not also essential when planning the teaching session to consider the communication tasks that need to be addressed? For instance, the communication challenge of offering choices to patients with breast cancer between lumpectomy and mastectomy is an issue that is known to affect postoperative psychological morbidity (Fallowfield *et al.* 1990). We need to become more adept at introducing relevant communication (process) issues into our content teaching.

Similarly, in our dedicated communication sessions, it is important not to neglect relevant content and perceptual issues. A family practice resident who omits to ask a young female patient with cystitis whether her symptoms are related to sexual intercourse may do so for one of two reasons. Embarrassment may get in the way of knowledge – the focus of the session might then be the communication issue of attempting to discover a way to ask sensitive questions in such embarrassing situations. Alternatively, the resident may not know of the link between intercourse and recurrent urinary tract infections and the focus of the session should then legitimately move to content rather than process.

In the above examples, the teaching sessions described have a major focus on either communication or knowledge and perceptual skills. Our task is to ensure that important complementary issues are not omitted. Balance is again the key.

THE INTEGRATIVE COURSE

We turn now to another approach to combining content, process and perceptual skills in which an entire course is deliberately planned to integrate and place emphasis on all three. We describe this course in some detail as it provides an excellent illustration of problem-based learning and skills integration in practice.

The Integrative Course is an essential component of Calgary's undergraduate medical programme. It consists of two problem-based learning courses that run for two and a half weeks, each unopposed by anything else in the overall medical curriculum. These courses are designed specifically to integrate the clinical skills of communication, physical examination and problem solving with each other and with the learners' expanding knowledge base of medical–technical information. Although this course is designed for undergraduates, the integrated approach can be equally useful with residents and in CME.

Small groups led by expert facilitators have the opportunity to interact with well over 20 simulated patients, each of whom presents with cross-system problem(s). Each small group of six to eight students has three or more hours per day, working with the same facilitator, to work through a number of these simulated cases, with exploration of one case lasting up to four days. Results of patients' investigations, including slides of ECGs, X-rays, CAT scans, etc., are available whenever students request them. Patients' complete 'charts' are available for the facilitator so that even if the problem is not in his area of specialization, he has at his fingertips all the necessary data for the case, including full details of past and present history, progress and outcomes, difficulties, suggested communication challenges, a list of resource people who might be called on to assist with the case, etc. A variety of communication issues are also introduced through these simulations, e.g. culture, gender, communicating with patients over multiple visits, third-party interviews, age, breaking bad news to patients, death and dying, bereavement, chronic and acute care, communication with medical colleagues and dealing with trauma.

Each simulation begins with the group observing as one student initiates the interview with the patient, gathers information about problems and starts to build a relationship. Physical examination may be performed at this point or the interviewer may first return to the group to discuss information obtained or missed so far, to consider what to include on physical examination, to generate and discuss hypotheses and eventually produce differential diagnoses. A list of learning issues, self-identified areas of lack of knowledge that the group feels would help their decision making or understanding, are also produced with the guidance of the facilitator.

The group continues problem solving and planning 'next steps' or else breaks to research learning issues or knowledge gaps which need to be worked through before they can continue. Learners divide up these learning issues and present their findings to the group in the following session.

Subsequent 'appointments' are made with the simulated patient so that learners can practise all aspects of explanation and planning. The Integrative Course is an excellent opportunity for undergraduates to experiment with these skills in a safe context. They have protected time to work through the medical facts about a situation or illness first. They then need to translate their knowledge into the world of the patient, giving information and translating the jargon that they have used in discussion within the group into a language that the patient can understand and accept. The individual student who gives information to the simulated patient is not put on the spot about his own factual knowledge as he is working on behalf of the group to impart their combined knowledge; the group can therefore concentrate on the communication skills and issues themselves.

Coordinating communication with other medical skills coursework and evaluation

Another strategy for integrating communication is to coordinate communication coursework and evaluation expressly with other components of the curriculum which aim to develop clinical skills.

Communication programme directors can enhance coordination and integration by encouraging directors of other courses and evaluations to include communication as an overlaid focus in their programmes and, in return, offering to overlay other courses' content in the communication course or evaluation. For example, invite nephrologists in the renal course to send patients to the communication course whom students can interview, or develop standardized patient cases which focus on problems discussed in the renal course; or check with clerkship directors to see if any of their oral examinations might evaluate communication process skills in addition to checking the content of the histories that students take. Ask physical examination course directors what they are teaching about communication with patients during the physical examination; work with them to develop OSCE stations which include communication process skills during both history and physical examination stations. Collaborate with human development, paediatrics or geriatrics courses to set up opportunities for students to interact with real or standardized patients who are children, elders or family members involved in their care. These efforts have the double benefit of making communication more visible and ensuring its status across disciplines.

A more formal way to accomplish integration is to house the communication curriculum administratively within a medical skills programme, formally bringing together into one administrative structure courses and evaluations on:

- communication
- physical examination
- ethics
- culture, health and illness
- medical informatics and technology

- well man and woman
- well physician
- evidence-based practice
- integrative courses.

This approach has recently been adopted in the undergraduate programme at the University of Calgary Faculty of Medicine and is described more fully in Appendix 1.

SECTION 2: HOW DO WE ASSESS LEARNERS' COMMUNICATION SKILLS?

Whether we like it or not, evaluation often drives the curriculum – what is evaluated gets taught and learned (Newble and Jaeger 1983; Westberg and Jason 1993; Pololi 1995; Southgate 1997).

Evaluation:

- motivates students to learn: unfortunately, students focus their energy on passing examinations necessary for their survival often to the point of neglecting other activities that would be more useful to their careers
- legitimizes the importance of the subject to students: unless a subject is assessed, students may not perceive it as an essential requirement for clinical practice but a soft subject of marginal importance
- encourages the acceptance of the subject by otherwise sceptical faculty staff: once a subject has been legitimized by becoming part of certifying evaluation, it becomes more readily accepted as a bona fide element of mainstream clinical education.

Clearly, if evaluation is such a potent force for establishing a subject within the overall curriculum, we must give careful thought to this aspect of the communication programme and use its potential to push the programme forward. If we embrace evaluation as an integral part of the teaching and learning process and convince learners and administrators to do the same, we are more likely to:

- devise evaluations that actually drive learning forward appropriately
- establish and extend the scope of the communication programme
- obtain the funding necessary for both evaluations and the programme itself.

Formative and summative assessment

Two distinct types of assessment are important components of well-designed communication curricula.

Formative assessment

Formative assessment is informal, ongoing assessment that forms an integral part of the teaching and learning process. It tends to take place during the course itself and to be the responsibility of both facilitators and the learning group.

The intention of formative assessment is to guide and foster learning under conditions that are non-judgemental and non-threatening. It has the potential to support the learner, improve the quality of teaching and enhance learning itself. Formative assessment provides opportunities for discovering problem areas or weaknesses without incurring academic penalty and with the promise of further help, guidance and action to rectify deficiencies (Rolfe and McPherson 1995).

A particular aim of formative assessment is to encourage honest and open self-assessment, for learners to feel free to admit and discuss their own difficulties. Learners need to feel able to express rather than hide problems so that they can receive constructive help in rectifying deficiencies and so that teachers can personalize their educational planning to meet the needs of each individual student. In much of traditional medical education, the culture of learning is judgemental and punitive and encourages learners to hide rather than to admit their deficiencies. Learners need to feel confident and supported by a well-motivated teacher to benefit from formative assessment (Ende *et al.* 1983; Knowles 1984; McKegney 1989; Westberg and Jason 1993).

Ongoing feedback to learners is an integral part of teaching methods employed in communication work and constitutes the primary formative assessment process. Experiential skills-based teaching, as described in the earlier chapters of this book, encompasses the concept of formative assessment to a much higher degree than traditional teaching methods.

Space can also be made within the course for periodic and slightly more formal formative assessment of learners to discuss progress so far and establish further learning needs. These regular reviews enable both the facilitator and learner to make appropriate mid-course corrections.

Summative or certifying assessment

Summative assessment occurs at preordained critical points and determines which learners move forward, which require further work and, ultimately, which pass and fail formal certification. Course organizers, faculty committees, licensing bodies and regional or national health authorities tend to take responsibility for setting these evaluations.

In contrast to formative assessment, summative assessment is typically based on information gathered at the end of a learning experience. As traditionally applied, feedback to learners is provided in simple judgements of pass, fail or grades and there is usually little potential for learning from the evaluation itself.

While in an ideal system formative assessment would be the major determinant of learners' efforts for self-improvement, in reality learners know that ultimate success or failure is dependent on passing certifying assessments. Learners therefore direct their attention preferentially towards activities that enable them to pass summative assessments and often ignore activities that appear to them not to be immediately relevant to that goal. It is therefore essential that those responsible for the summative evaluation system and who in effect control students' learning are mindful of the effects of their evaluations on the educational programme as a whole.

First, communication skills must be included in certifying assessments, even if such skills are more difficult to quantify and assess than lower levels of learning such as the recall of facts or technical skills. Unless complex higher order learning such as communication skills are assessed, learners will not consider it important to study these essential subjects (Westberg and Jason 1993).

Second, certifying evaluations should be matched to the learning objectives of the communication skills curriculum: these evaluations should be based on explicit published objectives which reflect the goals and philosophy of the communication course. The skills to be learned and assessed must be overtly stated to validate both the course and the assessment. Learners and teachers need to be aware of these objectives so that the assessment process can be seen to be directly related to learning within the communication curriculum.

Third, the methods of evaluation should mirror the methods of instruction. The methods used in summative assessment should not just measure the correct items of learning (content validity) but should measure them in a way that encourages learners to work and study for examinations using the methods of learning employed in the communication curriculum itself (consequential validity) (Holsgrove 1997). Unless this is done, learner behaviour may change in the opposite direction to that intended by the faculty or the course director (Newble and Jaeger 1983). Therefore, if direct observation is employed in both learning and formative assessment, it should be used in summative assessment as well. Similarly, the same instruments of assessment used in formative assessment should also be used in summative assessment. In fact, the only difference between formative and summative assessment should be the intent of the assessment, not the methods used. Learners should be entirely familiar with assessment methods and instruments before they reach summative assessment (Kurtz and Heaton 1987; Kurtz 1989).

In ongoing programmes with periodic certifying assessments, planning must include provision for both remediation and re-evaluation of learners who are unsatisfactory or who repeatedly demonstrate incompetence. Assessment is best thought of as a further component of helical learning: remediation followed by reassessment enables learners to take their next steps forward. Finding adequate facilitator and learner time for these processes is essential.

Working with learners who need remediation requires few special skills. It is, however, a time to be particularly adept in applying the facilitation techniques and models presented throughout this book. If remediation is required because of patient complaints over time or if emotional instability is a possibility, it is important to involve professionals who can determine whether personal problems or underlying psychiatric illness are at issue. If this is the case, assistance other than remediation may be more appropriate.

The framework and skills of the *Calgary–Cambridge observation guide* provide an excellent starting point for defining the objectives of both the communication curriculum and the evaluation process and for standardizing the instruments used in both formative and summative assessment.

Who does the actual assessments?

External examiners or experts, course facilitators, real and simulated patients, peers and even the learner who is under assessment may serve as evaluators for summative or formative assessment (Kurtz and Heaton 1987; Stillman *et al.* 1990a; Heaton and Kurtz 1992b; Westberg and Jason 1993; Farnill *et al.* 1997). Whatever the form of assessment used, establishing the evaluation's validity and reliability is important as is the provision of training for evaluators. Though peer and especially self-assessment carry less weight where they are used in certifying situations, they are of considerable value in formative assessment (Jolly *et al.* 1994). In fact, self-assessment is a vital step in formative assessment, as we describe in Chapter 5, in relation to experiential communication skills teaching sessions. There is an enormous difference between the learner who can appreciate that he has a difficulty and the learner who is unaware that he has a problem. The ability to self-assess is a prerequisite for becoming a life-long learner in independent clinical practice (Hays 1990).

What are you trying to assess?

A good starting point for designing assessments in the communication curriculum is to decide what you are trying to assess. The framework at the beginning of this chapter again proves useful.

Focuses of learning and assessment

First, are you designing evaluations that assess:

- knowledge
- competence
- performance or
- outcomes?

The educational level of the learner affects which of these can be attempted, but in our view, assessment of communication skills in medicine is relatively useless if it evaluates only knowledge, i.e. whether learners 'know about' the skills involved. Knowledge and understanding of the basic concepts of communication skills in the consultation are important and there is a place for including items on communication skills in written knowledge tests, not least to validate the importance of this subject to learners. But although evaluations of this sort can be performed inexpensively with paper and pencil tests, they do not assess the ability of the learner to use communication skills in practice. That goal requires evaluation of competence at least and, where possible, performance and outcome. While each of these categories provides indirect evidence of knowledge, knowledge alone offers little insight into the other three. Most evaluations of learners focus on competence (possible at all levels of medical education) and performance (possible at residency and CME levels) (Norman *et al.* 1985; Rethans *et al.* 1991).

Broad categories of skills

A second, important consideration is which communication skills you want to evaluate:

- content

- process or
- perceptual.

Content skills have to do with how accurate and complete the information is that is gathered from and given to patients.

Process skills include the core skills on our guide and the way they are used to initiate, gather information, build relationships, talk to patients during the physical examination, explain and plan, close the consultation and deal with communication challenges.

Perceptual skills have to do with problem solving, with ideas regarding hypotheses and problem lists, differential diagnoses and interpretation, as well as the handling of emotions and attitudes (the patient's and one's own).

Specific communication issues

Third, do you want to include assessment of how students deal with specific communication issues relevant to the context of your course, such as breaking bad news or working with patients from another culture or communicating with a depressed or psychotic patient?

What are the objectives of summative evaluation?

1 *Certification.* While the prime purpose of summative assessment of communication is the certification of learners, there are practical reasons for summative evaluations to include the following two additional objectives which can extend the scope of the communication programme and the value of the assessment.

2 *Teaching and learning* (as in detailed descriptive feedback, review and refinement, remedial work, built-in tutorials and even introduction of new material). In our view, summative evaluations can and should double as effective learning exercises that teach and reinforce even as they assess (Kurtz and Heaton 1987; Heaton and Kurtz 1992a). As the father of one of our colleagues says: 'You can't fatten a pig just by weighing it'. Summative assessment provides an excellent opportunity not only to determine the 5% who fail but also to benefit both them and the 95% who pass. By making evaluation an integral part of the communication curriculum, time is used in the most cost-effective manner. Practical assessments of communication and other clinical skills are costly and time intensive; if at all possible, use should be made of the availability of teaching staff, standardized patients and videotape for learning as well as evaluation. We find it useful for certifying evaluation to occur some weeks after the official end of coursework, thereby extending the curriculum without finding any 'extra' time and giving learners an opportunity to revive their communication training and take one more turn around the helix.

3 *Integration* (of communication with other clinical skills and knowledge base). Evaluations can be planned to assess jointly physical examination, medical problem-solving skills, knowledge, issues such as ethics and culture, and communication skills. This not only

makes assessment more efficient but extends students' and faculty's perceptions of the importance and value of communication as applied to actual patient problems and to their everyday work (Kurtz and Heaton 1987; Vu *et al*. 1992).

What form should assessments take?

Objective standardized clinical evaluation

Increasingly, summative assessment of competence and/or performance relies on some form of objective, standardized clinical evaluation (OSCE) using simulated patients (Harden and Gleeson 1979; Stillman and Swanson 1987; Langsley 1991; Grand 'Maison *et al*. 1992; Vu *et al*. 1992; Klass 1994; Vu and Barrows 1994; Pololi 1995). This form of evaluation can be constructed to meet all three objectives listed above.

The methodology of the OSCE fits well with the concept that the method of evaluation should mirror the method of instruction. The OSCE is an entirely logical extension of how we teach communication. Learners are assessed by direct observation of their ability to communicate with simulated patients in a standardized evaluation setting that is as close as possible to true life and in the context of situations or problems that learners will encounter in real medical practice. Simulated patients are trained so that they can give consistently accurate, standardized portrayals of specific cases and communication challenges, much as they would do in learning settings. Simulators can be real patients, learners role playing patients, evaluators role playing patients, 'matched' patients, volunteers from the community or actors.

Usually the evaluation consists of multiple stations, each presenting a different case or sometimes following one case across several stations. These may, for example, portray the original visit, a follow-up to give results of investigations, discuss diagnosis and treatment alternatives and then a third visit which in real life might have happened days or weeks later when complications developed. Evaluators watch the consultation(s) between learner and standardized patient live or on videotape and write comments on or score evaluation instruments that document the skills to be learned and assessed.

In a method pioneered in Calgary to incorporate teaching and learning into the assessment process, pairs of students actually take part with an evaluator in the very review of the learners' videotapes that comprises the certifying assessment procedure. By incorporating peer and self-evaluation and by discussing and contrasting two interviews with the same simulated patient as performed by the two different students, the assessment can take the form of a mini-tutorial to correct difficulties on the spot even if overall performance is rated as satisfactory (Heaton and Kurtz 1992*a,b*). Discussion of what works, what does not and what might be done to improve the interview occurs as the assessment proceeds. Students have an opportunity to see how peers deal with the same situation. The assessment becomes an ideal opportunity to correct problems, try out alternatives and reinforce and deepen skills.

The third objective of summative evaluation, integration, can be served by:

- constructing a communication case that also tests specific medical technical knowledge
- including physical examination as part of the history-taking station
- following a communication station with one requiring learners to conduct a physical examination relevant to the case

- providing learners with results of investigation and physical examination findings and asking them to interpret the findings given the history they have just taken
- integrating ethics and communication by selecting cases where learners deal with an ethical problem such as obtaining informed consent during the consultation.

OSCE examinations require a great deal of energy and time for students and examiners in addition to funding for simulated patients and possibly for examiners and administrative staff. Just as in coursework itself, OSCEs should be videotaped whenever possible as videotape is such an invaluable aid to assessment. Videotape can be reviewed at any time so the communication examiner does not need to be present during the consultation itself. Evaluators can replay any part of the evaluation at will to catch non-verbal behaviour or check out a first impression. Learners can review their tapes later or participate in the video review of their own tapes and those of other learners, as described above. Videotape also provides unarguable evidence of what happened during an evaluation, thus helping to avoid or resolve appeal problems (Heaton and Kurtz 1992b).

OSCEs are now widely used in certifying examinations in both Canada and the USA. They have become an established part of many medical schools' undergraduate and residency programmes (Vu et al. 1992; Anderson et al. 1994), have been used in provincial examinations for licensing family physicians (Grand 'Maison et al. 1992) and have begun to be introduced into national licensing examinations such as the Education Commission on Foreign Medical Graduates and the National Board of Medical Examiners (Langsley 1991; Klass 1994; Morrison and Barrows 1994). They are increasingly, although less commonly, used in the UK and Australasia (Newble and Wakeford 1994; Bingham et al. 1996). Considerable effort has been made to research the validity, reliability and feasibility of using standardized patients and OSCEs in certifying evaluations (van der Vleuten and Swanson 1990; Case and Bowmer 1994; Vu and Barrows 1994).

Other forms of assessment

An alternative approach to using simulated patients in certifying assessment is the use of video recordings of real consultations. Here, a series of consultations with real patients who present routinely to the clinic is videotaped with full patient consent and submitted by the learner for certifying assessment. This method is clearly more suitable for residency and CME than undergraduate training.

How the videotape is prepared will significantly influence whether competence or performance is assessed. For example, in the recently introduced summative assessment of minimal competence of UK general practice residents and the more stringent UK Membership of the Royal College of General Practitioners (MRCGP) examination, it has been decided to concentrate on competence (Conference of Postgraduate Advisors in General Practice 1995; RCGP 1996). Residents are allowed to submit consultations of their choosing that demonstrate their competence over a range of problems: the evaluation assesses 'can they do it?' not 'do they usually choose to do it?'. There is still ongoing discussion about issues of feasibility, cost, reliability and validity, particularly in relation to global versus detailed skills and competencies (Campbell et al. 1995a; Campbell and Murray 1996; Pereira Gray et al. 1997; Rhodes and Wolf 1997).

To come nearer to assessing performance, residents or practising physicians would need to submit tapes of many consecutive consultations with assessors choosing randomly from the material presented. Another approach to assessing performance for practising doctors and residents is to send simulated patients to the clinic unannounced and for the simulator to assess the clinician's performance: doctors are informed that the simulated patient will be coming within a specified time period and full consent is obtained (Burri *et al.* 1976; Norman *et al.* 1985; Rethans *et al.* 1991). A third approach currently being pilot-tested in Canada involves several of a physician's patients and combines videotape analysis with self-administered paper and pencil instruments which assess the perceptions of both patient and physician regarding their consultation (Stewart 1997).

What formats are available for feedback from both formative and summative evaluations?

Three continua describe the potential formats for evaluation that are available:

quantitative	qualitative
evaluative feedback	descriptive feedback
number scores, good/bad	'here's what I see'
global	detailed

Feedback forms themselves include:

- numbers-only rating scales
- numbers with explanatory comments attached for each question
- detailed check-lists with ratings of
  - pass/fail or
  - satisfactory (yes)/satisfactory but with significant performance deficiency ('yes, but' or 'see me')/unsatisfactory (no)
- rating scales or check-lists with space to write in comments
- comments only with no ratings given.

Our observation guides, as presented in Appendix 2, are an example of a way to structure feedback and formative assessment based on descriptive comments only. By adding columns for satisfactory, satisfactory but with significant performance deficiency, and unsatisfactory and adapting (or deleting) some items, we have used the same guide for certifying evaluations. The guide then becomes a check-list with ratings and comments for evaluation, and the basis for concrete, descriptive feedback to students and student self or peer assessment during video review (Heaton and Kurtz 1992b). Results can be quantified if necessary by assigning numbers to the three columns or adding a five-point, Likert-type unacceptable to exceptional scale (Turnbull *et al.*, research in progress).

Using a few global ratings for items such as 'ability to relate to patient' or 'interpersonal skills, scored by checking off a box or a Likert scale, was once the accepted norm for assessment of communication abilities. These were certainly simple to use and took little time to administer but unfortunately were vague and difficult for examiners and learners to interpret or learn from. These approaches did help draw attention to communication as a legitimate clinical skill but progress in research and assessment has given us much better and more detailed and specific alternatives.

For both formative and summative assessment, we therefore advocate formats on the right-hand-side of the continua that enable specific and detailed assessment of skills to be made and choose feedback forms or evaluation instruments with room for written comments to provide descriptive feedback to learners. In this way, we can encourage teaching and learning to be incorporated in the assessment process. We also encourage using the same form for both formative and summative assessments so that learners know exactly what skills or attitudes they are expected to be able to perform and so that they can follow their own progress (or regression) over time.

A number of different marking schedules, rating scales, check-lists with specific criteria and set scenarios in which key facets are identified have been developed both for OSCEs and videotaped consultations (Cox and Mulholland 1993; Bingham *et al.* 1994, 1996; Fraser *et al.* 1994; Rashid *et al.* 1994).

An excellent new resource on assessment is the *Evaluation of communication assessment tools* (Stewart and Boon 1997). This document describes in grid format some 15 patient satisfaction tools, 15 education tools (formative and summative assessment) and 26 research tools. Information is collated for each tool under the following headings: description, number of items, internal reliability, validity (concurrent, construct, predictive, face), use in practice/cancer care setting, possible use for self-assessment, and special notes.

9

The wider context

Introduction

In Chapter 8 we explored how to structure a communication skills curriculum in practice: we examined the important basic issues in curriculum design and saw how they pertained to all three levels of medical education. Here, we take a broader view and consider how we can develop the communication skills curriculum in the wider context of medical education as a whole. How do we promote the further development and acceptance of communication curricula within medical education? What key issues need to be addressed to enable communication programmes to become an established component of mainstream education throughout undergraduate, residency and continuing medical education? What barriers prevent communication from taking its place as an essential core subject at the centre of the medical curriculum? What resources can we draw on as we move to overcome these barriers? And what are the challenges for communication curricula in the years to come?

In this chapter we explore three related issues:

1 *promoting the further development and acceptance of communication curricula within medical education as a whole.* How can we:
   - find adequate time and resources for communication training in an already crowded curriculum?
   - coordinate the communication curriculum at all levels of medical education?
   - ensure the status of communication training across all specialties?
2 *enhancing facilitator training.* How can we:
   - enhance facilitators' own communication skills?
   - increase their knowledge base about communication skills, theory and research?
   - improve their communication teaching and facilitation skills?
   - maximize the status and reward of undertaking such teaching?
3 *looking to the future – where next?*
   - what are the domains of communication in health care beyond the doctor–patient consultation?
   - where are we now in the development of communication curricula and where do we go from here?

Promoting the further development and acceptance of communication curricula within medical education

What have been the blocks to progress in establishing effective communication skills teaching in medicine and what ways can we suggest to overcome these difficulties?

Finding adequate time and resources for communication training in an already overburdened curriculum

Finding adequate time for communication training is a major issue. All we have said so far in this volume suggests that if we wish to do justice to communication skills teaching and to achieve substantial and long-lasting changes in learners' communication skills, we need to dedicate significant time to the communication unit. The concepts of 'curriculum not course', 'helical rather than linear learning' and 'structured and organized communication skills teaching' all point towards a curriculum running throughout the medical course as a whole and requiring curriculum time on which there will no doubt be many other conflicting demands.

One example of an undergraduate programme which has put these concepts into practice is the communication curriculum at the University of Calgary's Faculty of Medicine. Initiated in the 1970s within Calgary's newly forged progressive medical school, the communication programme has gradually increased from a starting point of 16 hours dedicated time to its current standing of 45 hours of self-contained course time plus substantial additional time within other medical skills courses and clerkships. Appendix 1 describes the programme in more detail. Other medical schools in North America and Europe also currently devote considerable time and resources to communication teaching and learning. This pioneering work has established a historical precedent that benefits us all. It makes available a number of concrete resources which course developers and facilitators can draw upon:

- established programmes and approaches to teaching, learning and facilitator training which can serve as templates for developing programmes
- resource material, including videotapes, simulated patient cases, evaluation tools and designs, published journal articles and books, handouts, course outlines
- human resources with networks, conferences and journals for connecting; colleagues with experience and know-how who even at a distance can help resolve problems and share insights and strategies
- a strong research and conceptual base
- greater advocacy for and acceptance of communication teaching in medicine than has ever been the case before.

Because of the time and energy these resources can save, it is likely today to take less time to establish quality programmes than in the past. Yet like their predecessors, medical educators wishing to develop communication programmes still face two important challenges. First, they have to find money and resources in a hostile economic climate (Preston-White and McKinley 1993). Second, they are faced with having to gain acceptance for communication skills teaching in already established and crowded curricula (Sleight 1995). Not surprisingly, this can prove difficult as other disciplines and vested interests fight for their corner within the institution. So what can we do to encourage institutions to embrace the concept of communication skills training and to help them find adequate time and resources to do this subject justice?

USING THE PRESSURE FROM PROFESSIONAL MEDICAL BODIES
ON OUR MEDICAL INSTITUTIONS

Over the last two decades there has been increasing pressure from professional medical bodies throughout the world to improve the training and evaluation of doctors in communication skills. Medical institutions are feeling the force of this pressure as it is converted gradually from benign exhortation to more threatening formative evaluation of medical schools themselves and increasingly now to mandatory requirement. For example, in 1995, the bodies responsible for accrediting medical schools in Canada (Committee on Accreditation of Canadian Medical Schools) and the USA (Liaison Committee on Medical Education) both accepted statements requiring specific instruction and evaluation of communication skills as standards of accreditation (Barkun 1995). Groups which oversee residency training in these countries are moving toward similar requirements. At the same time, central bodies responsible for the national evaluation of learners are incorporating assessment of communication into their certifying examinations (Langsley 1991; Klass 1994; Morrison and Barrows 1994; Conference of Postgraduate Advisors in General Practice 1995; RCGP 1996). Medical institutions are becoming aware of the need to establish effective communication skills teaching to enable their learners to pass these national evaluations.

Simultaneously, medical schools are being asked to reduce the factual burden on learners as the potential knowledge base of medicine increases exponentially year by year. They are being encouraged to change the medical school curriculum to focus more thoroughly on certain core skills and areas of learning (of which communication is one) while providing a series of options for learners to choose from in less essential subjects (General Medical Council 1993; Metz *et al.* 1994; World Federation for Medical Education 1994).

In the face of such pressure to change, the committed communication skills programme 'salesman' may be received with open arms. Medical school authorities may be aware of what they are expected to do but still not know how to do so in practice. Communication skills teaching is a relatively new subject and most doctors in positions of authority will have had little, if any, personal experience of such teaching in their own training. They often have little understanding of how communication skills are taught. This situation represents both an opportunity and an obstacle to progress. While the authorities may embrace your willingness to establish a course, they may well not understand that communication skills teaching is different, that it requires a helical approach and that it must be spread throughout the medical curriculum. It is important to have facts and research evidence about communication teaching and learning at hand if we wish to convince others to provide the time and resources to establish effective communication skills programmes.

RIDING THE BACK OF OTHER INNOVATIONS IN MEDICAL EDUCATION

Other moves are afoot in medical education that offer opportunities for the communication programme director. Increasingly, medical schools are moving from a traditional to a problem-based curriculum. Problem-based learning offers considerable overlap with communication skills training methods and provides an ideal opportunity to extend the communication curriculum. What could be more problem based than a simulated patient case which learners work through over time, moving from information gathering to problem solving, then to investigating knowledge gaps and learning opportunities, and later returning to the simulated patient to explain findings and plan further care? The Integrative Course at the University of Calgary, described in Chapter 8, provides just such opportunities for learners. As problem-based learning becomes established in medical schools, communication skills programme directors can offer considerable help as their institutions struggle to put these new learning methods into practice.

Look for places where you can help solve dilemmas that learners or the curriculum committee have already discovered (e.g. lack of integration of knowledge with skills; failure of learners to apply skills in real settings that they seemed to possess in courses and in examinations; uncertainties about how to teach and assess skills). Look for ways to bring in innovations like the use of video work, OSCEs or simulated patients that might solve problems in other aspects of the programme while at the same time improving the communication curriculum.

Moves to combine clinical and preclinical training in medical schools and to make medical education more community based also offer opportunities to the communication director – each time the curriculum is thrown up in the air, the opportunity to promote communication skills within the system increases.

GETTING THE HEAVYWEIGHTS ON BOARD

Communication skills programmes must have the direct support of those in positions of authority. Without the active backing of deans within your institution or directors of your programmes, you will be facing an uphill struggle to achieve worthwhile change. Moreover, it is important that those in positions of power understand and are in sympathy with the concepts that underlie communication teaching. They may need winning over to your wish to extend communication teaching and to the teaching methods that need to be employed. Meetings to explain your position, discussions of what you have to offer the institution in relation to, say, reducing medico-legal complaints or increasing patient *and* doctor satisfaction, invitations to existing courses, clarity and specificity with respect to the skills and issues your curriculum will teach and the provision of well-reasoned literature may reap the benefit of providing your course with the support of those who can make things happen and sanction the necessary financial investment.

The availability of external funding is often needed to tip the balance and obtain the backing of those you need. Increasingly, pharmaceutical companies are providing financial resources for communication programmes which they see as important not only in securing drug compliance but also in raising their profile as ethical players in the health market (Carroll 1996). Similarly, improving the communication skills of doctors has a high standing in the public's eye and financial backing may well be available from private and charitable donations.

It is also important to obtain the support of champions and opinion leaders within your institution, those who command the respect of staff as a whole and who will provide your programme with positive affirmation during formal and informal discussion throughout the school. There is a considerable danger that much of our work can be undone by poor role modelling and lack of support from practising physicians. Clinicians who themselves have received little education in this field, may not value this aspect of their work and therefore not demonstrate in their own practice the skills that are being taught to juniors nor support changes to extend communication skills teaching within the institution. These negative messages can be countered by the endorsement of respected opinion leaders within the medical community.

Bringing in external experts from established centres of excellence can help influence those in positions of power to extend the communication curriculum. Organizations of those interested in communication skills teaching in medicine now exist throughout the world, such as the American Academy on Physician and Patient in the USA, the Bayer Institute for Health Care Communication in the USA and Canada, the Canadian Breast Cancer Initiative and the Medical Interview Teaching Association in the UK. Consider organizing visiting lectures and invite key players to attend. Organize a symposium to which gatekeepers, opinion leaders and external experts are invited to discuss the rationale for communication training, the research supporting it and the actions of similar groups who have already put such programmes into effect. Sponsors for such efforts can be found within local institutions, in national or state/provincial government health agencies, private foundations, pharmaceutical companies and health-related associations such as cancer societies.

MOTIVATING THE DOUBTERS

If faced with a seemingly insurmountable gap between your aspirations and the commitment of those around you in positions of power and influence, what else can you do to persuade such doubters to buy in? Here, we return to the material that we presented in Chapter 1 of this book. In your efforts at persuasion, present communication as:

- a core clinical skill as important as the physical examination
- a vital component of clinical competence as indispensable as knowledge, problem-solving ability and the physical examination
- leading to increased accuracy, efficiency and supportiveness and not just being nice
- a science with 25 years of accumulated theoretical and research evidence that has delineated the skills of effective communication and their relationship to improved health outcomes.

To convince doubters of the need to run communication skills programmes, we have to do more than extol the virtues of patient centredness. This cuts little ice with the unconverted. The really important selling point is that communication skills programmes actually enable learners to become more effective doctors clinically. There is no doubt that it is the prospect of improved clinical performance that interests doubters who otherwise view communication skills as an add-on extra of little clinical benefit.

Once the communication programme is established, a head of steam is created that encourages doubters to come on board. For example, the use of simulated patients in formal certifying examinations to test learners' communication skills enables the integrated assessment of communication, knowledge and other clinical skills in one reproducible setting. Not only is this a highly efficient approach to evaluation but it also leads to doctors who are assessing learners' skills in their parent subject being asked to rate learners' communication skills as well. Coming face to face with a marking grid that includes summarizing or eliciting information about the patient's perspective can act as a potent stimulus for interest and learning.

OFFERING PROGRAMME EFFICIENCIES

Many of the strategies that we outlined in Chapter 8 to integrate communication with other clinical skills offer efficiency savings that can be used to obtain more teaching time in the communication unit. These strategies include overlaying communication in other courses, incorporating other clinical skills within the communication programme (e.g. teaching the content of the clinical interview and physical examination), teaching ethics via the communication programme, initiating an integrative course to combine communication and problem-based learning and coordinating combined evaluations with other clinical skills. For instance, teaching the content and the process of the medical interview within one setting is not only educationally superior to teaching them separately in different units with different teachers, it is also more efficient. Offering to take on such traditional content teaching within the communication unit is a means of obtaining further time from the overall curriculum.

SHAMELESSLY EMPLOYING THE STICK AND THE CARROT WITH LEARNERS

Much as we would prefer otherwise, it is often the stick of compulsory assessment rather than selfless enquiry that motivates learners to engage in teaching programmes (Newble and Jaeger 1983). Given the nature of human beings, the carrot of financial inducement can act as an equally effective motivator. This is especially true in CME where most education is voluntary and the limiting factor in introducing new educational areas into the curriculum is not competition for curriculum time but learner commitment. Here, the stick of re-accreditation and the carrot of CME credits and insurance premium reductions seem to act as potent stimuli to learners (Carroll 1996).

Motivating learners in these ways can add pressure to medical institutions to improve teaching: there is no doubt, for example, that compulsory summative assessment in communication skills in British general practice residency training has led to a clamour for improved teaching from learners. Communication skills teaching has benefited as collusion between poorly motivated learners and poorly skilled underconfident teachers has melted away. In turn, communication skills programmes have gained extra credibility and resources.

Coordinating the communication curriculum at all levels of medical education

At present, coordination of communication curricula between undergraduate, postgraduate and CME is one of the weakest links in our efforts to improve communication in medicine. As undergraduate communication programmes vary tremendously, postgraduate programmes cannot rely on incoming residents' prior learning, much less on what they have retained. Residency programmes vary even more both within and between specialties and many offer no formal communication component at all. CME therefore inherits a group of learners with disparate communication expertise.

Nonetheless, a number of experiments to increase coordination are under way. Many administrators and course organizers recognize the need for such collaboration and are working towards it within their own institutions. In some locations, committees of interested individuals have formed which include representations from each level. Joint discussion and planning within these groups encourage cross-fertilization of ideas and coordination of efforts.

Mandates from accrediting or licensing bodies at all three levels are making communication training and evaluation a compulsory requirement. These mandates promote coordination – new communication programmes are appearing and their directors are contacting directors of existing programmes for ideas and advice. As more and more learners leave well-run undergraduate programmes they are in a position to influence and participate in the ongoing development at residency and CME levels.

Local, regional, national and international conferences, such as the biannual Ottawa Conference on Teaching and Assessment of Clinical Skills, are of major importance. Initiatives, such as the Canadian Breast Cancer Initiatives Professional Education Strategy, which bring together interested parties can also have a significant impact on coordinating education and promoting research on communication education. Joint training is of considerable value. For instance, the Bayer Institute for Health Care Communication (USA and Canada) provides training courses to prepare facilitators from all three levels of medical education to lead workshops and provides participants with a common and in-depth understanding of how to teach communication in medicine.

An increasing range of medical journals is accepting and soliciting articles on communication teaching and research. Books, such as this one, promote coordination and contribute to the establishment of conceptual common ground across levels; instruments such as the *Calgary–Cambridge observation guide* provide a common set of skills for teaching and evaluation programmes at all levels.

Ensuring the status of communication training as a bona fide clinical skill across all specialties

Traditionally, communication has been taught primarily by general practitioners and psychiatrists without the input of other specialist groups. This can give an inappropriate message to learners about the bona fide nature of communication as a clinical skill central to all fields of medicine. If specialists are not involved in teaching communication, learners may conclude that it is not of importance in specialist care. How then can we involve specialists in the communication programme? Firstly, we can invite them to be facilitators in our courses. It is essential to extend the facilitation of this subject to as wide a group of specialists as possible to promote communication teaching throughout the medical school structure and to give it wider recognition within the medical school as a whole. Similarly, exposing specialists to overlays of communication within other courses and to evaluations in which communication is integrated with other clinical skills serves to advertise the importance of communication and the methods with which it is taught.

Virtually all of the suggestions and strategies mentioned in this book contribute toward ensuring the status of communication as a bona fide skill across all specialties. In Canada, considerable progress has been made on this issue over the past few years, thanks in large part to the strategies listed above under 'Coordinating the communication curriculum at all levels of medical education'. These particular strategies may be a useful starting point for dealing with this issue elsewhere.

Enhancing facilitator training

In our experience, facilitator training is of central importance in establishing successful communication programmes. In addition to setting up a programme for our learners, we have to take one step backwards and consider how to train our facilitators as well. We ignore this step at our peril. Facilitators need training to enable them to become skilled and comfortable in their teaching. Yet often this issue receives scant attention in our efforts to develop communication curricula. Perhaps programme directors find it difficult to ask willing facilitators who may be very experienced in their own field of study (be it medicine, psychology or communication studies) to undergo such training or take the time that it involves. But in our experience, facilitators often feel at sea in the milieu of communication teaching and value any input that we can provide.

Why is training for facilitators so important?

COMMUNICATION SKILLS TEACHING REQUIRES A LARGE NUMBER OF FACILITATORS

Communication skills teaching is labour intensive. Experiential group work, essential to this teaching, requires one facilitator for every four to eight learners. One-to-one teaching requires even more facilitators. Furthermore, good communication skills teaching is an ongoing process; many inputs are required of the numerous facilitators involved. In a typical medical school there may be from 70 to a few hundred students per year, each requiring multiple teaching sessions in small groups. A large number of competent facilitators are therefore required.

COMMUNICATION SKILLS TEACHING IS DIFFERENT

As we have discussed, communication skills facilitation in medicine is different from other forms of teaching. It has its own subject matter and methodology. Communication is more closely bound to learners' self-concept and esteem than other areas of teaching. And, despite evidence to the contrary, learners may still come with a perception that communication is more a matter of personality or attitudes than of skills and cannot be taught.

We cannot assume that previous experience of teaching or medical practice is all that is required to teach this unique subject. It simply does not follow that skills or knowledge in other areas of medicine equip you to teach communication.

COMMUNICATION SKILLS TEACHING IS DIFFICULT

Communication skills teaching also requires considerable knowledge and skill. Facilitators need to know about three major areas:

1 the 'what' of communication skills teaching
2 the 'how' of communication skills teaching
3 the 'how' of small-group or one-to-one facilitation.

Facilitators may need considerable help with knowing 'what' to teach, including:

- the skills that are worth teaching
- a way to structure those skills into a coherent and memorable whole
- the research and theoretical evidence that validates the use of specific communication skills
- the overall breadth of the communication skills curriculum.

The 'how' of communication skills teaching includes the specific teaching methods for ana-lysing and providing feedback on a consultation as well as the more widely applicable core skills of small-group or one-to-one facilitation which are required to maximize participation and learning. Many doctors have little experience of working in a supportive group, let alone leading it, and benefit from focused training to help them develop the skills required. We can-not assume that teachers brought up in traditional medical education understand the prin-ciples of supportive group work and even if they do, they may well have received little instruction on how to put their understanding into practice.

ADDRESSING FACILITATORS' OWN COMMUNICATION SKILLS WITH PATIENTS

In coaching doctors about how to facilitate communication skills learning, we often have the added complication of having to address their own physician–patient communication skills as well as their teaching skills. Many potential facilitators belong to a generation of doctors who received little or no teaching of communication skills in their own education. We cannot there-fore make the assumption that facilitators have any better grasp of the subject matter than their learners nor that they are necessarily any better at communication in their own practice of medicine. We described this situation in Chapter 2 as 'the blind leading the partially sighted'. Even when doctors are excellent communicators, they may well have never analysed what they themselves do and so may be unable to teach it. Unless we help our facilitators to feel comfortable with their own abilities to communicate and to analyse quite what it is that constitutes good communication, they may have considerable difficulties teaching and modelling the appropriate skills to learners. Like a good tennis coach or piano teacher, a communication teacher needs both to be reasonably proficient and to understand what com-prises proficiency to teach others well!

Enhancing facilitators' skills

Facilitators face three agendas in their training:

1 enhancing their own personal communication skills
2 increasing their knowledge base about communication skills theory and research
3 enhancing their communication teaching and facilitation skills.

Time is clearly a major issue. First, there are many skills and a large amount of knowledge for facilitators to assimilate. It is simply not possible to do justice to all three areas unless time is allocated to the process and the project is appropriately resourced. There is no reason to be-lieve that facilitators will take any less time to explore their own communication skills than any other group of learners in CME. And having completed that task, the process of learning how to teach the subject will take a similar length of time. Second, not only will facilitators' training in their own communication skills need to be helical and ongoing but also their training in facilitation skills will need to follow the same path of regular review, reiteration and increasing complexity.

This may seem too daunting to the programme director: 'How can I possibly resource such facilitator training programmes; how can I ever get my facilitators to free up the necessary time to leave their busy practices?'. Nevertheless we strongly recommend that these difficult issues be tackled rather than swept under the carpet as without attention to facilitator training, communication skills programmes will fail to achieve their true potential. Two separate surveys of Canadian medical schools (in 1994 and 1996) confirm this assertion: both identified lack of trained faculty as the number one barrier to improving undergraduate communication curricula (Cowan *et al.* 1997). Of course, it does not all need to be done at once and programmes for learners can be established alongside ongoing programmes for facilitators. But facilitator training does need to keep moving along: helical learning works best when the gaps between training sessions are not so large that all learning is forgotten.

Examples of facilitator training programmes

Before looking at how to overcome the obstacles that stand in the way of establishing comprehensive facilitation training programmes, it is helpful to look at three different approaches to facilitator training.

EXAMPLE 1

This first programme was developed in the East Anglian region of England to train medical facilitators to teach communication to a high standard in both residency and CME in postgraduate general practice. It is based on two components:

1 *Materials and methods.* A manual on communication skills teaching initially provided facilitators with the theoretical knowledge and research evidence to validate individual communication skills and a detailed explanation of specific teaching methods (Silverman *et al.* 1996*a*). This book and its companion volume have now become the major print resources for the training programme.

2 *Ongoing experiential training.* Just as you cannot teach communication skills by didactic methods alone, so you cannot teach communication skills teaching without experiential methods of observation, feedback and rehearsal. Facilitators need print resources that they can use both to increase their knowledge base and to refer to repeatedly when they are back home continuing their own skill development and teaching. However, written material is not enough by itself. Facilitators have to move from understanding what the appropriate facilitation skills are to learning in practice how to incorporate these skills into their teaching. They need to practise and refine their communication skills facilitation and require constructive feedback to develop their teaching skills.

The facilitator training programme therefore offers an initial three-day intensive residential course to address facilitators' own communication skills *and* start the process of examining their teaching skills. This is followed by regular follow-up days every three months in which the group reconvenes for a whole day to:

- continue their own communication skills learning
- share their experiences of teaching
- advance their helical learning by observing each other teach in practice through either role play or pre-recorded videotapes of their actual teaching in their home programmes.

In the early stages, the programme enables participants to experience the process of learning doctor–patient communication skills in an experiential small-group setting. Simultaneously, they learn about communication skills teaching by experiencing the process at first hand and observing established facilitators. As the programme progresses, the emphasis gradually moves from learners' own communication with patients to their teaching skills, with increasing observation, feedback and rehearsal of their teaching rather than of their doctor–patient skills. However, both processes continue to occur to enable helical reiteration and repetition to flourish.

The individuals in the group are committed to participating in ongoing training. The same group follows through the programme together, forming a team or cohort which over time provides each individual with a base of trusted colleagues who support each other in their efforts, provide a stable forum for discussing teaching problems they encounter and stimulate each other's thinking and skill development.

EXAMPLE 2

A second programme uses facilitator training of doctors paired with other health professionals as a strategy for improving communication with patients in eight interlinked cancer centres simultaneously (Cowan and Laidlaw 1997). Sponsored by the Ontario Cancer Treatment and Research Foundation (OCTRF), this programme works from the premise that a team will be more influential in improving communication skills within the institution than an individual working alone. The OCTRF sent a pair of interested individuals (one doctor, one non-doctor staff member) from each centre to a five-day training course for facilitators run by the Bayer Institute for Health Care Communication. Each pair then spearheaded communication training for staff within their own centres via workshops and subsequent follow-up with activities such as communication rounds. In these workshops the learners were mixed groups comprising doctors, nurses, pharmacists, psychologists, radiotherapists, administrators, residents, medical students, receptionists and clerical staff. This multifaceted group were then in a position to support each other's efforts at communicating with patients and to influence overall communication within the cancer centre as a whole.

The facilitators from all the centres meet as a group every three months to support each other, compare notes and pursue planning and ongoing problem solving. Within a year, 380 participants (of whom 49 were physicians and 48 residents) had taken part in 31 workshops and follow-up. Not surprisingly, if the chief executive officer of the institution attended, that influenced everyone else's participation noticeably.

EXAMPLE 3

A third set of strategies involves on-the-job training (Kurtz 1985). These strategies do not constitute a well-developed training programme but course directors may find them useful in supporting facilitators where formal training programmes cannot be mounted immediately.

- *Resource materials for independent study:* core documents describing objectives of the overall course and individual sessions (e.g. the *Calgary–Cambridge observation guide*); resource materials such as this book and its companion volume; computerized medical communication databases such as the Dalhousie Medcom Collection (Laidlaw 1997); brief sessions to orient facilitators to these materials and share ideas for getting started
- *Direct coaching and assistance:* telephone calls; being available before, during and after teaching sessions; informing facilitators about techniques that other groups are trying; modelling teaching skills as a drop-in or invited participant; offering workshops to course facilitators; arranging communication skills workshops and other meetings to enhance skills
- *Enlisting others to assist:* teaching simulated patients to model effective feedback; pairing inexperienced with outstanding, experienced facilitators; suggesting ideas for teaching and learning to students
- *Miscellaneous:* encouraging facilitators to stay with the course to develop a core of experience over time; requiring a formative but written evaluation of learners part way through the course to open the door for discussion of problems or questions; holding strategy sessions with facilitators and administrators to develop options for providing more elaborate facilitator training programmes.

Maximizing the status and reward of undertaking such teaching

If facilitator training programmes are to flourish, we must look carefully at how to overcome the obstacles that stand in the way of their implementation. The overriding problems in facilitator training are time and money. In many contexts, doctors volunteer their teaching time for free and few mechanisms exist to recompense them for their own ongoing training in teaching. Doctors can face considerable potential loss of earnings by giving up their practices for the requisite time for both teaching and training. How can we change the current climate in which education is so often undervalued?

IMPROVING THE STATUS OF TEACHING IN GENERAL

One of the key obstacles in securing financial support for facilitator training relates to the second-class status accorded to teaching as opposed to research or administration within academic institutions. For many years, the apprenticeship model of medical training has predominated – special skills in teaching have not been valued. Financial rewards in the university academic environment have closely followed research output or administrative skills.

Too little credit has been given to teaching excellence. And yet teaching is a key responsibility in academic life. It is therefore politically important to assist in the current movement to increase the status of teaching. Only when education is truly valued will it be adequately rewarded, financially or otherwise. Fortunately, moves are already afoot in this direction. Increasingly, for instance, residency training is moving to an educational rather than a service model. Political moves have helped this process. In the UK, half of the money for the salaries of residents in all specialties has been moved from the hospital to the postgraduate dean's budget. This single change gives the dean improved power in securing the status of residency education and increased responsibility for ensuring that the teaching process is of high quality. In many university settings, significant policy shifts now credit a focus on teaching, developing curricula, creating resources for teaching, publishing about teaching and undertaking personal skill development which contributes to teaching excellence as routes toward merit and promotion. These shifts are an important advance toward securing the status of teaching.

OBTAINING OTHER REWARDS FOR TRAINED FACILITATORS

There are several other ways to secure rewards for those who become communication skills facilitators. Both teaching and the training undertaken to learn to teach can be credited as part of CME. For instance, in the British system of postgraduate education allowance (PGEA) for established general practitioners, family doctors purchase their CME to qualify for a substantial financial allowance. Not only does running a communication course under this scheme provide free PGEA points for anyone teaching on the course, it also entitles facilitators to claim fees for their services. CME credit works in the same way in Canada and we have been successful in gaining CME credits for doctors who facilitate in undergraduate courses. Family practice and other specialists in Canada and the United States have received CME credits for undertaking training to improve their ability to communicate with patients and to teach communication. Medical insurance premium reductions are available for those with communication skills training within several states of the USA. This of course also applies to those trained to facilitate these courses. So either directly or indirectly, communication teaching and personal skill enhancement can open the door to financial and educational benefits.

A no less important reward on offer to those involved in communication teaching is the improvement in their own practice of medicine: we are pleased to report that this still seems to be the prime motivator of many of our facilitators! Gratifyingly, the satisfaction of helping learners to improve their communication skills also overrides many financial and practical difficulties to create its own very special reward.

Looking to the future – where next?

One more issue remains: what will the well-rounded communication curricula of the future include? To answer this question, we take a comprehensive look at the various domains which fit under the heading of communication in medicine, assess where we are now in developing communication curricula and anticipate possibilities for the future.

Domains of communication in medicine

Improving communication in medicine clearly involves more than just the skills of one-to-one doctor–patient communication. What about:

- third-party consultations where family or significant others are involved
- communication between doctors or between doctors and other health professionals

- the needs of a team of health care professionals attempting to coordinate their interactions with patients (and often patients' family members)
- communicating at a distance through the telephone or telemedicine
- how computers in the office affect our communication with patients
- developing patients' communication skills in health care?

If we take this broader picture into account and think in terms of the future, what areas do we need to consider? What domains contribute to effective communication in health care?

Interestingly, Kurtz (1996) in North America and Weatherall (1996) in Britain answered these questions in presentations at separate conferences with almost identical lists of domains. We combine their efforts here by listing the domains and providing examples which describe each area more fully. The list is a template for present and future planning.

1 **Physician–patient interaction:**
   - accuracy, efficiency, supportiveness
   - information gathering
   - explanation and planning, decision making, negotiation
   - relationship building
   - counselling and psychosocial therapy
   - third-party communication (patient's family, significant others)
   - enhancing patients' ability to communicate with health professionals and within the system
2 **Communication issues:**
   - culture
   - ethics
   - gender
   - special needs patients (elderly, young, challenged, low literacy)
   - prevention, motivation to change
   - dealing with feelings
   - confrontation
   - breaking bad news, death and dying
   - addiction
   - malpractice
3 **Communication with self:**
   - thought processes
   - clinical reasoning and problem solving
   - attitudes
   - feelings
   - reflection/self-evaluation
   - dealing with stress and tension, personal flexibility
   - handling mistakes
   - handling failures
   - biases
4 **Communicating with other professionals:**
   - colleagues in medicine
   - colleagues in nursing and the allied health professions
   - health care teams (formal and informal; talking within the team and with patients)
   - administrators

- researchers (directly and through the literature)
- making presentations and lectures, discussion leadership

5 **Communicating at a distance:**
- telephone
- medical records (written and computerized), fax, letters
- computer-assisted interviewing and consults
- telemedicine (including transmission of images, vital signs, etc.)
- databases, websites, electronic networks (from libraries to dialogue groups)
- newspapers, popular magazines, scientific journals

6 **Health promotion via mass media, communicating with the public:**
- pamphlets, brochures, posters
- radio and television campaigns
- advertising
- 'edutainment' (health-related audio/videotapes, CDs and video games)
- public speaking
- talking to the press

7 **Communicating with 'the system' (government, community, hospital, etc.):**
- influencing health policy
- talking with government, community and agency representatives
- influencing and coping with change

Where are we now and where do we go from here?

To the best of our knowledge, no existing programme fully covers all these seven domains and certainly it would be counter-productive to try to implement a programme with the intent of focusing on all these areas at once.

We have chosen to focus our own approach primarily on the first domain: the skills of physician–patient communication. We also place significant emphasis on the two other domains which influence physician–patient communication most immediately, namely communication issues and communication with self. At present, however, our approach has little direct emphasis on the remaining domains, 4 to 7.

A FIRST TIER IN COMMUNICATION PROGRAMME DEVELOPMENT

Our current emphasis on the first three domains makes sense for the following reasons:

- both patient and physician groups have expressed a desire to improve physician–patient communication – at present there is widespread interest and advocacy in this area
- a substantial research base concerning physician–patient communication has been developed in the past 25 years – we know considerably more about how to improve this domain than we are currently achieving in practice
- improving physician–patient communication skills sets the stage for improvement across the board – it makes sense to focus on this domain first because the skills that constitute effective doctor–patient communication are core skills that can be adapted to improving communication in all the other domains.

One aspect of the first domain which receives too little attention in many programmes, including our own, is communication with third parties, for example:

- parents of children
- family members of elderly patients or significant others assisting in their care
- individuals involved in the care of chronically ill patients
- companions of people with impaired sight or hearing
- interpreters assisting individuals who speak languages different from the physician's.

Improving our programmes in these areas is a logical next step.

A second, underdeveloped aspect of communication between doctors and patients that is gaining rapid momentum is the improvement of *patients'* own understanding of their interactions with doctors and others in the health care system and the development of their own communication skills within the consultation. Researchers have shown that when patients participate in training about how to talk with their doctors and take a more active part in the consultation, outcomes improve (see Chapter 5 of our companion volume). Doctors have an active role to play here, either by contributing directly toward this effort or by supporting others working in this area. Health care organizations and professional groups are encouraging progress (e.g. the Canadian Breast Cancer Initiatives Professional Education Strategy and the International Communication Association Division of Health Communication). The work of King *et al.* (1985) in Britain and Pantell *et al.* (1986), Bernzweig *et al.* (1997) and Korsch and Harding (1997) in the United States includes valuable material written for patients in this regard that doctors would clearly benefit from reading too. This is an area that requires further attention in communication programmes of the present and the future.

A SECOND TIER IN COMMUNICATION PROGRAMME DEVELOPMENT

Domains 4 and 5 might logically become part of a second tier of development effort: with few exceptions the skills involved in physician–patient communication apply equally well to communicating with professional colleagues. Communication with other professionals and communicating at a distance are everyday aspects of any doctor's practice. They are increasingly important in health care, a trend that is likely to be even more pronounced in the coming years. We know less about these domains from the literature; both of these areas are ripe for research. Residency and CME levels are the logical places in which to develop these domains.

A THIRD TIER IN COMMUNICATION PROGRAMME DEVELOPMENT

Finally, domains 6 and 7 might become part of a third tier of development in which some physicians choose to participate. While it is unlikely that every physician will need to develop these skills, mass communication is an area where medical professionals are becoming increasingly involved. Also evident is the need for some physicians to engage in speaking to small and large groups about issues of health and health promotion. With all the changes that health care is undergoing, more physicians may need to develop expert skills in influencing health policy through communication with groups and individuals, private and public agencies, within their own institutions and communities and at the provincial/state and national levels. And clearly, everyone would benefit from developing the skills needed to cope with change.

References

American Board of Pediatrics (1987) Teaching and evaluation of interpersonal skills and ethical decision-making in pediatrics. *Pediatrics.* **79**: 829–33.

Anderson MB, Stillman PL and Wang Y (1994) Growing use of standardised patients in teaching and evaluation in clinical medicine. *Teaching and Learning in Med.* **6**: 15–22.

Arborelius E and Bremberg S (1992) What can doctors do to achieve a successful consultation? Video-taped interviews analysed by the 'consultation map' method. *Fam Pract.* **9**: 61–6.

Association of American Medical Colleges Panel on the General Professional Education of the Physician and College Preparation for Medicine (1984) *Physicians for the twenty-first century: The GPEP report.* Association of American Medical Colleges, Washington D.C.

Avery JK (1986) Lawyers tell what turns some patients litiginous. *Med Malpract Rev.* **2**: 35–7.

Bain J and Mackay NSD (1993) Videotaping general practice consultations. [Letter] *BMJ.* **307**: 504–5.

Baker SJ (1955) The theory of silences. *J Gen Psychol.* **53**: 145.

Bandura A (1988) *Principles of behavior modification.* Holt, Rinehart and Winston, New York.

Barkun H (1995) Personal communication. Former Executive Director of the Association of Canadian Medical Colleges.

Barrows HS (1987) *Simulated (standardised) patients and other human simulations.* Health Sciences Consortium, Chapel Hill, NC.

Barrows HS and Abrahamson S (1964) The programmed patient: a technique for appraising clinical performance in clinical neurology. *J Med Educ.* **39**: 802–5.

Barrows HS and Tamblyn RM (1981) *Problem based learning: an approach to medical education.* Springer Publishing House, New York.

Bass LW and Cohen RL (1982) Ostensible versus actual reasons for seeking pediatric attention: another look at the parental ticket of admission. *Pediatrics.* **70**: 870–4.

Beckman HB and Frankel RM (1984) The effect of physician behaviour on the collection of data. *Ann Intern Med.* **101**: 692–6.

Beckman HB and Frankel RM (1994) The use of videotape in internal medicine training. *J Gen Intern Med.* **9**: 517–21.

Beckman HB, Markakis KM, Suchman AL *et al.* (1994) The doctor–patient relationship and malpractice. *Arch Intern Med.* **154**: 1365–70.

Beisecker A and Beisecker T (1990) Patient information-seeking behaviours when communicating with doctors. *Med Care.* **28**: 19–28.

Berg JS, Dischler J, Wagner DJ *et al.* (1993) Medication compliance: a health care problem. *Ann Pharmacotherapy.* **27**: 3–22.

Bernzweig J, Takayama JI, Phibbs C *et al.* (1997) Gender differences in physician–patient communication: evidence in pediatric visits. *Arch Ped Adol Med.* **151**: 586–91.

Bertakis KD (1977) The communication of information from physician to patient: a method for increasing patient retention and satisfaction. *J Fam Pract.* **5**: 217– 22.

Bingham E, Burrows PJ, Caird GR *et al.* (1994) Simulated surgery: a framework for the assessment of clinical competence. *Educ for Gen Pract.* **5**: 143–50.

Bingham L, Burrows P, Caird R *et al.* (1996) Simulated surgery – using standardized patients to assess clinical competence of GP registrars – a potential clinical component of the MRCGP examination. *Educ for Gen Pract.* **7**: 102–11.

Bird J and Cohen-Cole SA (1983) Teaching psychiatry to non-psychiatrists. 1. The application of educational methodology. *Gen Hosp Psychiat.* **5**: 247–53.

Bowman FM, Goldberg D, Millar T *et al.* (1992) Improving the skills of established general practitioners: the long-term benefits of group teaching. *Med Educ.* **26**: 63–8.

Briggs GW and Banahan BF (1979) *A training workshop in psychological medicine for teachers of family medicine.* Handouts 1–3. Therapeutic communication. Society of Teachers of Family Medicine, Denver, CO.

Brod TM, Cohen MM and Weinstock E (1986) *Cancer disclosure: communicating the diagnosis to patients – a videotape.* Medcom Inc, Garden Grove, CA.

Burri A, McCaughan K and Barrows HS (1976) The feasibility of the use of simulated patients as a means to evaluate clinical competence of practicing physicians in a community. *Proceedings of the 15th Conference on Research in Medical Education,* San Francisco, CA.

Butler C, Rollnick S and Stott N (1996) The practitioner, the patient and resistance to change: recent ideas on compliance. *Can Med Assoc.* **154**(9): 1357–62.

Byrne PS and Long BEL (1976) *Doctors talking to patients.* Her Majesty's Stationery Office, London.

Callaway S, Bosshart DA and O'Donnell AA (1977) Patient simulators in teaching patient education skills to family practice residents. *J Fam Pract.* **4**: 709–12.

Campbell LM and Murray TS (1996) Summative assessment of vocational trainees: results of a three-year study. *Br J Gen Pract.* **46**: 411–4.

Campbell LM, Howie JGR and Murray TS (1995*a*) Use of videotaped consultations in summative assessment of trainees in general practice. *Br J Gen Pract.* **45**: 137–41.

Campbell LM, Sullivan F and Murray TS (1995*b*) Videotaping of general practice consultations: effect on patient satisfaction. *BMJ.* **311**: 236.

Carroll JG (1996) Medical discourse: 'difficult' patients and frustrated doctors. Paper presented at the Oxford Conference on Teaching about Communication in Medicine, Oxford. Bayer Institute for Health Care Communication, Inc.

Carroll JG and Monroe J (1979) Teaching medical interviewing: a critique of educational research and practice. *J Med Educ.* **54**: 498–500.

Carroll JG, Schwartz MW and Ludwig S (1981) An evaluation of simulated patients as instructors: implications for teaching medical interviewing skills. *J Med Educ.* **56**: 522–4.

Case S and Bowmer I (1994) Licensure and specialty board certification in North America: background information and issues. In *The certification and recertification of doctors* (eds D Newble, B Jolly and R Wakefield). Cambridge University Press, Cambridge.

Cassata DM (1978) Health communication theory and research: an overview of the communication specialist interface. In *Communication Yearbook* (ed BD Ruben). Transaction Books, New Brunswick, NJ.

Chugh U, Dillman E, Kurtz SM *et al.* (1993) Multicultural issues in medical curriculum: implications for Canadian physicians. *Med Teacher.* **15**: 83–91.

Coambs R, Jensen P, Hoa Her M *et al.* (1995) *Review of the scientific literature on the prevalence, consequences, and health costs of non-compliance and inappropriate use of prescription medication in Canada.* Pharmaceutical Manufacturers Association of Canada (University of Toronto Press), Ottawa.

Cohen-Cole SA (1991) *The medical interview: a three-function approach.* Mosby Year Book, St. Louis.

Cohen-Cole SA, Bird J and Mance R (1995) Teaching with role play – a structured approach. In *The medical interview* (eds M Lipkin Jr, SM Putnam and A Lazare). Springer-Verlag, New York.

Conference of Postgraduate Advisors in General Practice, Universities of the United Kingdom. (1995) *Summative assessment.* London.

Coonar AS, Dooley M, Daniels M *et al.* (1991)The use of role play in teaching medical students obstetrics and gynaecology. *Med Teacher.* **13**: 49–53.

Cowan DH and Laidlaw JC (1993) Improvement of teaching and assessment of doctor–patient communication in Canadian medical schools. *J Cancer Educ.* **8**: 109–17.

Cowan D and Laidlaw J (1997) Personal communication. Ontario Cancer Treatment and Research Foundation, Toronto, Ontario, Canada.

Cowan DH, Laidlaw JC and Russell L (1997) *Research report: results of two surveys regarding the teaching and evaluation of doctor/patient communication in Canadian medical schools.* (Submitted for publication.)

Cox A (1989) Eliciting patients' feelings. In *Communicating with Medical Patients* (eds M Stewart and D Roter). Sage Publications, Newbury Park, CA.

Cox J and Mulholland H (1993) An instrument for assessment of video tapes of general practitioners' performance. *BMJ.* **306**: 1043–6.

Craig JL (1992) Retention of interviewing skills learned by first-year medical students: a longitudinal study. *Med Educ.* **26**: 276–81.

Dance FEX (1967) Toward a theory of human communication. In *Human communication theory: original essays* (ed FEX Dance). Holt, Rhinehart and Winston, New York.

Dance FEX and Larson CE (1972) *Speech communication: concepts and behavior.* Holt, Rinehart and Winston, New York.

Davidoff F (1993) Medical interviewing: the crucial skill that gets short shrift. *ACP Observer.* **June**: 15.

Davis H and Nicholaou T (1992) A comparison of the interviewing skills of first- and final-year medical students. *Med Educ.* **26**: 441–7.

Descouteaux JG (1996) *Perceived need for communication skills training: implications for instructional design*. Poster presented at Annual Meeting of the Royal College of Physicians and Surgeons of Canada, Halifax, Nova Scotia (September).

DeVito JA (1988) *Human communication: the basic course* (4th edn). Harper & Row, New York.

DiMatteo MR, Hays RD and Prince LM (1986) Relationship of physicians' non verbal communication skill to patient satisfaction, appointment non-compliance and physician workload. *Health Psychol.* **5**: 581–94.

Egan G (1990) *The skilled helper: a systematic approach to effective helping*. Brooks/Cole, Pacific Grove, CA.

Eisenthal S and Lazare A (1976) Evaluation of the initial interview in a walk-in clinic. *J Nervous and Mental Disease.* **162**: 169–76.

Eisenthal S, Koopman C and Stoeckle JD (1990) The nature of patients' requests for physicians' help. *Academic Med.* **65**: 401–5.

Eleftheriadou Z (1996) Communicating with patients of different backgrounds. In *Communication skills for medicine* (eds M Lloyd and R Bor). Churchill Livingstone, Edinburgh.

Ende J, Kazis L, Ash AB *et al.* (1983) Measuring patients' desire for autonomy. *J Gen Intern Med.* **4**: 23–30.

Engler CM, Saltzman GA, Walker ML *et al.* (1981) Medical student acquisition and retention of communication and interviewing skills. *J Med Educ.* **56**: 572–9.

Evans BJ, Stanley RO, Burrows GD *et al.* (1989) Lecture and skills workshops as teaching formats in a history taking skills course for medical students *Med Educ.* **23**: 364–70.

Evans BJ, Stanley RO, Mestrovic R *et al.* (1991) Effects of communication skills training on students' diagnostic efficiency. *Med Educ.* **25**: 517–26.

Fallowfield LJ, Hall A, Maguire GP *et al.* (1990) Psychological outcomes of different treatment policies in women with early breast cancer outside a clinical trial. *BMJ.* **301**: 575–80.

Farnill D, Hayes SC and Todisco J (1997) Interviewing skills: self-evaluation by medical students. *Med Educ.* **31**: 122–7.

Ficklin FL (1988) Faculty and housestaff members as role models. *J Med Educ.* **63**: 392–6.

Finlay I and Dallimore D (1991) Your child is dead. *BMJ.* **302**: 1524–5.

Foreman KJ, Kurtz SM, Spronk BJ *et al.* (1996) Conflict as a positive tension. Chapter in unpublished project report. *Participatory education in cross-cultural settings*. Canada–Asia Partnership, Division of International Development, International Centre, University of Calgary, Canada.

Fraser RC, McKinley RK and Mulholland H (1994) Consultation competence in general practice: testing the reliability of the Leicester assessment package. *Br J Gen Pract.* **44**: 293–6.

Gask L, McGrath D, Goldberg D *et al.* (1987) Improving the psychiatric skills of established general practitioners: evaluation of group teaching. *Med Educ.* **21**: 362–8.

Gask L, Goldberg D, Lesser AL *et al.* (1988) Improving the psychiatric skills of the general practice trainee: an evaluation of a group training course. *Med Educ.* **22**: 132–8.

Gask L, Goldberg D and Boardman A (1991) Training general practitioners to teach psychiatric interviewing skills: an evaluation of group training. *Med Educ.* **25**: 444–51.

General Medical Council (1978) *Report of a working party of the Education Committee on the Teaching of Behavioural Sciences, Community Medicine and General Practice in Basic Medical Education*. GMC, London.

General Medical Council (1993) *Tomorrow's doctors: recommendations on undergraduate medical education.* GMC, London.

General Medical Council (1995) News review. London.

Gibb JR (1961) Defensive communication. *J Commun.* **3**: 142.

Gill PS and Adshead D (1996) Teaching cultural aspects of health: a vital part of communication. *Med Teacher.* **18**: 61–4.

Goldberg D, Steele JJ, Smith C *et al.* (1980) Training family practice doctors to recognise psychiatric illness with increased accuracy. *Lancet.* **2**: 521–3.

Goldberg D, Steele JJ, Smith C *et al.* (1983) *Training family practice residents to recognise psychiatric disturbances.* National Institute of Mental Health, Rockville, MD.

Gorden T and Burch N (1974) *TET: Teacher effectiveness training.* David McKay, New York.

Grand 'Maison P, Lescop J and Rainsberry P (1992) Large-scale use of an objective, structured, clinical examination for licensing family physicians. *Can Med Assoc J.* **146**: 1735–40.

Hadlow J and Pitts M (1991) The understanding of common terms by doctors, nurses and patients. *Soc Sci Med.* **32**: 193–6.

Hall JA, Roter DL and Katz NR (1988) Meta-analysis of correlates of provider behaviour in medical encounters. *Med Care.* **26**: 657–75.

Hampton JR, Harrison MJG, Mitchell JRA *et al.* (1975) Relative contributions of history-taking, physical examination and laboratory investigation to diagnosis and management of medical out-patients. *BMJ.* **2**: 486–9.

Harden RM and Gleeson F (1979) Assessment of clinical competence using an objective structured clinical examination. *Med Educ.* **13**: 41.

Hargie ODW and Morrow NC (1986) Using videotape in communication skills training: a critical review of the process of self-viewing. *Med Teacher.* **8**: 359–65.

Hays RB (1990) Content validity of a general practice rating scale. *Med Educ.* **24**: 110–16.

Heaton CJ and Kurtz SM (1992a) The role of evaluation in the development of clinical competence: no one ever fattened a pig just by weighing it. In *Proceedings of the International Conference on Current Development in Assessing Clinical Competence* (eds GR Hart and IR Hart), pp. 226–33. Heal Publications, Montreal.

Heaton CJ and Kurtz SM (1992b) Videotape recall: learning and assessment in certifying exams. In *International Conference Proceedings: Developments in Assessing Clinical Competence* (eds IR Hart and R Hardin), pp. 541–7. Heal Publications, Montreal.

Helfer RE (1970) An objective comparison of the pediatric interviewing skills of freshman and senior medical students. *Pediatrics.* **45**: 623–7.

Helfer RE and Levin S (1967) The use of videotape in teaching clinical pediatrics. *J Med Educ.* **42**: 867.

Helfer RE, Black M and Helfer M (1975a) Pediatric interviewing skills taught by non-physicians. *Am J Dis Child.* **129**: 1053–7.

Helfer RE, Black M and Teitelbaum H (1975b) A comparison of pediatric interviewing skills using real and simulated mothers. *Pediatrics.* **55**: 397–400.

Holsgrove G (1997) Principles of assessment. In *Teaching medicine in the community* (eds C Whitehouse, M Roland and P Campion). Oxford University Press, Oxford.

Hoppe RB (1995) Standardized (simulated) patients and the medical interview. In *The Medical Interview* (eds M Lipkin Jr, SM Putnam and A Lazare). Springer-Verlag, New York.

Hoppe RB, Farquhar LJ, Henry R *et al.* (1990) Residents' attitudes towards, and skills in, counselling using undetected standardized patients. *J Gen Intern Med.* **5**: 415–20.

Inui TS, Yourtee EL and Williamson JW (1976) Improved outcomes in hypertension after physician tutorials. *Ann Intern Med.* **84**: 646–51.

Irwin WG and Bamber JH (1984) An evaluation of medical students' behaviour in communication. *Med Educ.* **18**: 90–5.

Jason H and Westberg J (1982) *Teachers and teaching in US medical schools.* Appleton Century Crofts, Norwalk, CN.

Jason H, Kagan N, Werner A *et al.* (1971) New approaches to teaching basic interview skills to medical students. *Am J Psych.* **127**: 1404–7.

Johnson DW (1972) *Reaching out: interpersonal effectiveness and self-actualization.* Prentice-Hall, Englewood Cliffs, NJ.

Jolly B, Cushing A and Dacre J (1994) Reliability and validity of a patient-based workbook for assessment of clinical and communication skills. *Proceedings of the Sixth Ottawa Conference on Medical Education* (eds A Rothman and R Cohen). University of Toronto Bookstore, Custom Publishing, Toronto.

Joos SK, Hickam DH, Gordon GH *et al.* (1996) Effects of a physician communication intervention on patient care outcomes. *J Gen Intern Med.* **11**: 147–55.

Kahn GS, Cohen B and Jason HJ (1979) The teaching of interpersonal skills in US medical schools. *J Med Educ.* **54**: 29–35.

Kaplan SH, Greenfield S and Ware JE (1989) Assessing the effects of physician–patient interactions on the outcomes of chronic disease. *Med Care.* **27**: S110–27.

Kaplan SH, Greenfield S, Gandek B *et al.* (1996) Characteristics of physicians with participatory decision-making styles. *Ann Intern Med.* **124**: 497–504.

Kauss DR, Robbins AS, Abrass I *et al.* (1980) The long-term effectiveness of interpersonal skills training in medical schools. *J Med Educ.* **55**: 595–601.

Keller V and Carroll JG (1994) A new model for physician–patient communication. *Patient Education and Counselling.* **23**: 131–40.

Keller V and Kemp White M (1997) *Choices and changes: clinician influence and Patient Action workshop workbook.* Bayer Institute for Health Communication, West Haven, CT.

Kent CC, Clarke P and Dalrymple-Smith D (1981) The patient is the expert: a technique for teaching interviewing skills. *Med Educ.* **15**: 38–42.

Kindelan K and Kent G (1987) Concordance between patients' information preferences and general practitioners' perceptions. *Psychol Health.* **1**: 399–409.

King AM, Prkowski-Rogers LC and Pohl HS (1994) Planning standardised patient programmes: case development, patient training and costs. *Teaching and Learning in Med.* **6**: 6–14.

King J, Pendleton D and Tate P (1985) *Making the most of your doctor: a family guide to dealing with your GP.* Thames Television International, London.

Klass DJ (1994) High-stakes testing of medical students using standardised patients. *Teaching and Learning in Med.* **6**: 28–32.

Knowles MS (1984) *The adult learner – a neglected species.* Gulf, Houston, TX.

Koh KT, Goh LG and Tan TC (1991) Using role play to teach consultation skills – the Singapore experience. *Med Teacher.* **13**: 55–61.

Korsch BM and Harding C (1997) *The intelligent patient's guide to the doctor–patient relationship.* Oxford University Press, New York.

Korsch BM, Gozzi EK and Francis V (1968) Gaps in doctor–patient communication. *Pediatrics.* **42**: 855–71.

Kraan HF, Crijnen AA, de Vries MW *et al.* (1990) To what extent are medical interviewing skills teachable? *Med Teacher.* **12**: 315–28.

Kurtz SM (1975) *Physician non-verbal behavior and patient satisfaction in physician–patient interviews.* Doctoral dissertation, University of Denver, Colorado.

Kurtz SM (1985) On-the-job strategies for preceptor training. Paper presented at the International Communication Association Conference, Honolulu, May.

Kurtz SM (1989) Curriculum structuring to enhance communication skills development. In *Communicating with medical patients* (eds D Roter and M Stewart). Sage Publications, Newbury Park, CA.

Kurtz SM (1990) Attending rounds: a format and techniques for improving teaching and learning. In *Proceedings of the Third International Conference on Teaching and Assessing Clinical Competence* (ed W Bender), pp. 61–5. Groningen, The Netherlands.

Kurtz SM (1996) Collaboration in physician–patient communication: The Calgary–Cambridge approach. A paper presented to Communication in Breast Cancer – A Forum to Develop Strategies to Enhance Physician–Patient Communication. Sponsored by Health Canada's Canadian Breast Cancer Initiative: Professional Development Strategy. February 11–13, Calgary, Alberta.

Kurtz SM and Heaton CJ (1987) Coordinated clinical skills evaluation in the preclinical years: helical progression makes sense. In *Further developments in assessing clinical competence* (eds IR Hart and RM Hardin), pp. 172–84. Heal Publications, Montreal.

Kurtz SM and Heaton CJ (1995) Teaching and assessing information-giving skills in the communication curriculum. In *Proceedings of the Sixth Ottawa Conference on Medical Education* (eds AI Rothman and R Cohen), pp. 524–6. University of Toronto Bookstore, Custom Publishing, Toronto.

Kurtz SM and Silverman JD (1996) The Calgary–Cambridge observation guides: an aid to defining the curriculum and organising the teaching in communication training programmes. *Med Educ.* **30**: 83–9.

Laidlaw T (1997) *Dalhousie Medcom Collection.* Faculty of Medicine, Division of Medical Education, Dalhousie University, Nova Scotia.

Langsley DG (1991) Medical competence and performance assessment: a new era. *JAMA.* **266**: 977–80.

Larsen KM and Smith CK (1981) Assessment of non-verbal communication in the patient–physician interview. *J Fam Pract.* **12**: 481–8.

Levenkron JC, Grenland P and Bowley M (1987) Using patient instructors to teach behavioral counselling skills. *J Med Educ.* **62**: 665–72.

Levinson W (1994) Physician–patient communication: a key to malpractice prevention. *JAMA.* **272**: 1619–20.

Levinson W and Roter D (1993) The effects of two continuing medical education programs on communication skills of practicing primary care physicians. *J Gen Intern Med.* **8**: 318–24.

Levinson W and Roter D (1995) Physicians' psychosocial beliefs correlate with their patient communication skills. *J Gen Intern Med.* **10**: 375–9.

Levinson W, Stiles WB, Inui TS *et al.* (1993) Physician frustration in communicating with patients. *Med Care.* **31**(4): 285–95.

Ley P (1988) *Communication with patients: improving satisfaction and compliance.* Croom Helm, London.

Lipkin M Jr, Quill TE and Napedano RJ (1984) The medical interview: a core curriculum for residencies in internal medicine. *Ann Intern Med.* **100**: 277–84.

Lipkin M Jr, Kaplan C, Clark W *et al.* (1995) Teaching medical interviewing: the Lipkin model. In *The medical interview* (eds M Lipkin, SM Putman and A Lazare). Springer-Verlag, New York.

Littlewood R and Lipsedge M (1993) *Aliens and alienists: ethnic minorities and psychiatry.* Routledge, London.

McAvoy BR (1988) Teaching clinical skills to medical students: the use of simulated patients and videotaping in general practice. *Med Educ.* **22**: 193–9.

McKegney CP (1989) Medical education: a neglectful and abusive family system. *Fam Med.* **21**(6): 452–7.

McWhinney I (1989) The need for a transformed clinical method. In *Communicating with medical patients* (eds M Stewart and D Roter). Sage Publications, Newbury Park, CA.

Maguire P (1976) The use of patient simulation in training medical students in history-taking skills. *Med Biol Illus.* **26**: 91–5.

Maguire P and Faulkner A (1988a) Communicate with cancer patients. 1. Handling bad news and difficult questions. *BMJ.* **297**: 907–9.

Maguire P and Faulkner A (1988b) Improve the counselling skills of doctors and nurses in cancer care. *BMJ.* **297**: 847–9.

Maguire P and Rutter D (1976) History taking for medical students. 1. Deficiencies in performance. *Lancet.* **2**: 556–8.

Maguire P, Roe P, Goldberg D *et al.* (1978) The value of feedback in teaching interviewing skills to medical students. *Psychological Med.* **8**: 695–704.

Maguire P, Fairbairn S and Fletcher C (1986a) Consultation skills of young doctors. 1. Benefits of feedback training in interviewing as students persist. *BMJ.* **292**: 1573–6.

Maguire P, Fairbairn S and Fletcher C (1986b) Consultation skills of young doctors. 2. Most young doctors are bad at giving information. *BMJ.* **292**: 1576–8.

Maguire P, Faulkner A, Booth K *et al.* (1996) Helping cancer patients disclose their concern. *Eur J Cancer.* **32A**: 78–81.

Maiman LA, Becker MH, Liptak GS *et al.* (1988) Improving pediatricians' compliance-enhancing practices: a randomized trial. *Am J Dis Child.* **142**: 773–9.

Makoul G, Arnston P and Scofield T (1995) Health promotion in primary care: physician–patient communication and decision about prescription medications. *Soc Sci Med.* **41**: 1241–54.

Mansfield F (1991) Supervised role play in the teaching of the process of consultation. *Med Educ.* **25**: 485–90.

Martin E and Martin PML (1984) The reactions of patients to a video camera in the consulting room. *J RCGP.* **34**: 607–10.

Maynard DW (1990) Bearing bad news. *Med Encounter*. **7**: 2–3.

Mehrabian A and Ksionsky S (1974) *A theory of affiliation*. Lexington Books, DC Health and Co., Lexington, MA.

Meichenbaum D and Turk DC (1987) *Facilitating treatment adherence: a practitioner's guidebook*. Plenum Press, New York.

Metz JCM, Stoelinga GBA, Pels Rijcken-Van Erp Taalman Kip EH *et al.* (1994) *Blueprint 1994: Training of doctors in the Netherlands*. University of Nijmegen, The Netherlands.

Miller GE (1990) *Commentary on clinical skills assessment: a specific review*, pp. 48–51. National Board of Medical Examiners' 75th Anniversary, Philadelphia.

Miller GR and Steinberg M (1975) *Between people: a new analysis of interpersonal communication*. Science Research Associates, Chicago, IL.

Monahan DJ, Grover PL and Kalley R (1988) Evaluation of communication skills course for second year medical students. *J Med Educ*. **63**: 327–8.

Morrison LJ and Barrows HS (1994) Developing consortia for clinical practice examinations: the Macy project. *Teaching and Learning in Med*. **6**: 23–7.

Mumford E, Schlesinger HJ and Glass GV (1982) The effects of psychological intervention on recovery from surgery and heart attacks: an analysis of the literature. *AJPH*. **72**: 141–51.

Myers KW (1983) Filming the consultation – an educational experience. *Update*. **26**: 1731–9.

Newble D and Jaeger K (1983) The effect of assessments and examinations on the learning of medical students. *Med Educ*. **17**: 165–71.

Newble D and Wakeford R (1994) Primary certification in the UK and Australasia. In *The certification and recertification of doctors* (eds D Newble, B Jolly and R Wakeford). Cambridge University Press, Cambridge.

Norman GR (1985) Objective measurement of clinical performance. *Med Educ*. **19**: 43–7.

Norman GR, Neufield VR and Walsh A (1985) Measuring physicians' performances by using simulated patients. *J Med Educ*. **60**: 925–34.

Novack DH, Dube C and Goldstein MG (1992) Teaching medical interviewing: a basic course on interviewing and the physician–patient relationship. *Arch Intern Med*. **152**: 1814–20.

Novack DH, Volk G, Drossman DA *et al.* (1993) Medical interviewing and interpersonal skills teaching in US medical schools: practice, problems and promise. *JAMA*. **269**: 2101–5.

Orth JE, Stiles WB, Scherwitz L *et al.* (1987) Patient exposition and provider explanation in routine interviews and hypertensive patients' blood pressure control. *Health Psychol*. **6**: 29–42.

Pacoe LV, Naar R, Guyett PR *et al.* (1976) Training medical students in interpersonal relationship skills. *J Med Educ*. **51**: 743.

Pantell R, Lewis C, Bergman D *et al.* (1986) Improving medical visit process and outcome: results of a randomized control communication intervention. Paper and resources presented at International Conference on Doctor–Patient Communication, Centre for Studies in Family Medicine, University of Western Ontario (September).

Pendleton D, Schofield T, Tate P *et al.* (1984) *The consultation: an approach to learning and teaching*. Oxford University Press, Oxford.

Pereira-Gray D, Murray TS, Hasler J *et al.* (1997) The summative assessment package: an alternative view. *Educ Gen Pract.* **8**: 8–15.

Peterson MC, Holbrook J, VonHales D *et al.* (1992) Contributions of the history, physical examination and laboratory investigation in making medical diagnoses. *West J Med.* **156**: 163–5.

Pinder R (1990) *The management of chronic disease: patient and doctor perspectives on Parkinson's disease.* Macmillan Press, London.

Platt FW and McMath JC (1979) Clinical hypocompetence: the interview. *Ann Intern Med.* **91**: 898–902.

Pololi LH (1995) Standardised patients: as we evaluate so shall we reap. *Lancet.* **345**: 966–8.

Premi J (1991) An assessment of 15 years' experience in using videotape review in a family practice residency. *Acad Med.* **66**: 56–7.

Preston-White M and McKinley RK (1993) Teaching communication skills: funding required for teaching programmes. *BMJ.* **307**: 130.

Pringle M and Stewart-Evans C (1990) Does awareness of being video recorded affect doctors' consultation behaviour? *Br J Gen Pract.* **40**: 455–8.

Prochaska JO and DiClemente CC (1986) Towards a comprehensive model of change. In *Treating addictive behaviors* (eds R Miller and N Heather). Plenum Press, New York.

Putnam SM, Stiles WB, Jacob MC *et al.* (1988) Teaching the medical interview: an intervention study. *J Gen Intern Med.* **3**: 38–47.

Rashid A, Allen J, Thaw R *et al.* (1994) Performance-based assessment using simulated patients. *Educ Gen Pract.* **5**: 151–6.

Rethans JJ, Sturmans F, Drop R *et al.* (1991) Does competence of general practitioners predict their performance? Comparison between examination setting and actual practice. *BMJ.* **303**: 1377–80.

Rhodes M and Wolf A (1997) The summative assessment package: a closer look. *Educ Gen Pract.* **8**: 1–7.

Riccardi VM and Kurtz SM (1983) *Communication and counselling in health care.* Charles C Thomas, Springfield, IL.

Ridsdale L, Morgan M and Morris R (1992) Doctors' interviewing technique and its response to different booking time. *Fam Pract.* **9**: 57–60.

Roe P (1980) *Training medical students in interviewing skills.* M.Sc. thesis, University of Manchester.

Rogers CR (1980) *A way of being.* Houghton Mifflin, Boston, MA.

Rolfe I and McPherson J (1995) Formative assessment: how am I doing? *Lancet.* **345**: 837–9.

Rost KM, Flavin KS, Cole K *et al.* (1991) Change in metabolic control and functional status after hospitalisation. *Diabetes Care.* **14**: 881–9.

Roter DL (1997) Influencing health care outcomes through enhanced communications. Paper presented at Building Synergies in Communication: Linking Research and Practice. Conference of the Canadian Breast Cancer Initiative, Health Canada (February).

Roter DL and Hall JA (1987) Physicians' interviewing styles and medical information obtained from patients. *J Gen Intern Med.* **2**: 325–9.

Roter DL and Hall JA (1992) *Doctors talking with patients, patients talking with doctors.* Auburn House, Westport, CT.

Roter DL, Hall JA and Katz NR (1987) Relations between physicians' behaviour and analogue: patients satisfaction, recall and impressions. *Med Care*. **25**: 437–51.

Roter DL, Hall JA, Kern DE *et al.* (1995) Improving physicians' interviewing skills and reducing patients' emotional distress. *Arch Intern Med*. **155**: 1877–84.

Royal College of General Practitioners Membership Examination (1996) *Assessment of consulting skills workbook*. London.

Royal College of Physicians (1997) *Improving communication between doctors and patients*. RCGP, London.

Rutter D and Maguire P (1976) History-taking for medical students. 2. Valuation of a training programme. *Lancet*. **2**: 558–60.

Saebo L, Rethans JJ, Johannessen T *et al.* (1995) Standardized patients in general practice – a new method for quality assurance in Norway. *Tidsskrift for Den Norske Laegeforening*. **115**: 3117–19.

Sanson-Fisher RW (1981) *Personal communication*. Faculty of Medicine, University of Newcastle, New South Wales, Australia.

Sanson-Fisher RW and Poole AD (1978) Training medical students to empathize: an experimental study. *Med J Australia*. **1**: 473–6.

Sanson-Fisher RW and Poole AD (1980) Simulated patients and the assessment of students' interpersonal skills. *Med Educ*. **14**: 249–53.

Sanson-Fisher RW, Redman S, Walsh R *et al.* (1991) Training medical practitioners in information transfer skills: the new challenge. *Med Educ*. **25**: 322–33.

Schmidt HG (1983) Problem-based learning: rationale and description. *Med Educ*. **17**: 11.

Schulman BA (1979) Active patient orientation and outcomes in hypertensive treatment. *Med Care*. **17**: 267–81.

Schutz WC (1967) *Joy: expanding human awareness*. Holt, Rinehart and Winston, New York.

Seely JF, Jensen N, Kurtz SM *et al.* (1995) Teaching and assessing communication skills. *Ann RCPS Canada*. **28**(1): 33–6.

Servant JB and Matheson JAB (1986) Video recording in general practice: the patients do mind. *Br J Gen Pract*. **36**: 555–6.

Sharp PC, Pearce KA, Konen JC *et al.* (1996) Using standardized patient instructors to teach health promotion interviewing skills. *Fam Med*. **28**: 103–6.

Siegler M, Reaven N, Lipinski R *et al.* (1987) Effect of role-model clinicians on students' attitudes in a second-year course on the introduction to the patient. *J Med Educ*. **62**: 935–7.

Silverman JD, Draper J and Kurtz SM (1996a) *Teaching communication skills: an evidence-based manual for group work facilitators in vocational training and CME*. General Practice Office, NHS Executive, Anglia & Oxford, Cambridge.

Silverman JD, Kurtz SM and Draper J (1996b) The Calgary–Cambridge approach to communication skills teaching. 1. Agenda-led, outcome-based analysis of the consultation. *Educ Gen Pract*. **7**: 288–99.

Silverman JD, Draper J and Kurtz SM (1997) The Calgary–Cambridge approach to communication skills teaching. 2. The Set-Go method of descriptive feedback. *Educ Gen Pract*. **8**: 16–23.

Simpson MA (1985) How to use role play in medical teaching. *Med Teacher*. **7**: 75–82.

Simpson M, Buckman R, Stewart M *et al.* (1991) Doctor–patient communication: the Toronto consensus statement. *BMJ*. **303**: 1385–7.

Sleight P (1995) Teaching communication skills: part of medical education? *J Human Hypertension*. **9**: 67–9.

Southgate L (1993) *Statement on the use of video recording of general practice consultations for teaching, learning and assessment: the importance of ethical considerations*. RCGP, London.

Southgate L (1997) Assessing communication skills. In *Teaching medicine in the community* (eds C Whitehouse, M Roland and P Campion). Oxford University Press, Oxford.

Starfield B, Wray C, Hess K *et al.* (1981) The influence of patient–practitioner agreement on outcome of care. *AJPH*. **71**: 127–31.

Stewart J and D'Angelo G (1975) *Together: communicating interpersonally*. Addison-Wesley Publishing Company, Reading, MA.

Stewart MA (1984) What is a successful doctor–patient interview? A study of interactions and outcomes. *Soc Sci Med*. **19**: 167–75.

Stewart MA (1997) *Self-assessment and feedback on communication with patients*. Maintenance of Competence Program of the Royal College of Physicians and Surgeons of Canada and Disease Prevention Division of Health, Canada.

Stewart MA and Boon H (1997) *Evaluation of communication assessment tools*. Centre for Studies in Family Medicine, University of Western Ontario. Resource presented at Building Synergies in Communication: Linking Research and Practice. Conference of the Canadian Breast Cancer Initiative, Health Canada (February).

Stewart MA and Roter D (eds) (1989) *Communicating with medical patients*. Sage Publications, Newbury Park, CA.

Stewart MA, McWhinney IR and Buck CW (1979) The doctor–patient relationship and its effect upon outcome. *J RCGP*. **29**: 77–82.

Stewart MA, Belle Brown J, Wayne Weston W *et al.* (1995) *Patient-centred medicine: transforming the clinical method*. Sage, Thousand Oaks, CA.

Stewart MA, Belle Brown J, Donner A *et al.* (1997) *The impact of patient-centred care on patient outcomes in family practice*. Research report, Thames Valley Family Practice Research Unit, Ontario.

Stillman PL and Swanson DB (1987) Ensuring the clinical competence of medical school graduates through standardized patients. *Arch Intern Med*. **147**: 1049–52.

Stillman PL, Sabars DL and Redfield DL (1976) Use of paraprofessionals to teach interviewing skills. *Pediatrics*. **57**: 769–74.

Stillman PL, Sabars DL and Redfield DL (1977) Use of trained mothers to teach interviewing skills to first-year medical students: a follow up study. *Pediatrics*. **60**: 165–9.

Stillman PL, Burpeau-DiGregorio MY, Nicholson GI *et al.* (1983) Six years of experience teaching patient instructors to teach interviewing skills. *J Med Educ*. **58**: 941–6.

Stillman PL, Swanson DB, Smee S *et al.* (1986) Assessing clinical skills of residents with standardized patients. *Ann Intern Med*. **105**: 762–71.

Stillman P, Regan MB and Swanson DA (1987) Diagnostic fourth-year performance assessment. *Arch Intern Med.* **19**: 1981–5.

Stillman PL, Regan MB, Philbin M *et al.* (1990*a*) Results of a survey on the use of standardized patients to teach and evaluate clinical skills. *Acad Med.* **65**: 288–92.

Stillman PL, Regan MB and Swanson DB (1990*b*) An assessment of the clinical skills of fourth-year students at four New England medical schools. *Acad Med.* **65**: 320–6.

Svarstad BL (1974) *The doctor–patient encounter: an observational study of communication and outcome.* Doctoral dissertation, University of Wisconsin, Madison.

The Headache Study Group of The University of Western Ontario (1986) Predictors of outcome in headache patients presenting to family physicians – a one-year prospective study. *Headache J.* **26**: 285–94.

Thew R and Worrall P (In press) The selection and training of patient-simulators for the assessment of consultation performance in simulated surgeries. *Educ Gen Pract.*

Tuckett D, Boulton M, Olson C *et al.* (1985) *Meetings between experts: an approach to sharing ideas in medical consultations.* Tavistock, London.

Turnbull J, Kurtz SM, Blackmore G *et al.* (Research in progress) *The external validation of an assessment of communication skills.* University of Ottawa, University of Calgary, Medical Council of Canada.

van Dalen J, Zuidweg J and Collet J (1989) The curriculum of communication skills teaching at Maastricht Medical School. *Med Educ.* **23**: 55–61.

van der Vleuten C and Swanson D (1990) Assessment of clinical skills with standardised patients: state of the art. *Teaching and Learning in Med.* **2**: 58–76.

van Thiel J, Kraan HF and van der Vleuten CPM (1991) Reliability and feasibility of measuring medical interviewing skills: the revised Maastricht history-taking and advice check-list. *Med Educ.* **25**: 224–9.

Vu NV and Barrows H (1994) Use of standardised patients in clinical assessments: recent developments and measurement findings. *Educational Researcher.* **23**: 23–30.

Vu NV, Barrows H, Marcy M *et al.* (1992) Six years of comprehensive, clinical, performance-based assessment using standardized patients at the Southern Illinois University School of Medicine. *Acad Med.* **67**: 42–50.

Wackman DB, Miller S and Nunnally EW (1976) *Student workbook: increasing awareness and communication skills.* Interpersonal communication programmes, Minneapolis.

Waitzkin H (1984) Doctor–patient communication: clinical implications of social scientific research. *JAMA.* **252**: 2441–6.

Walton J, Duncan AS, Fletcher CM *et al.* (1980) *Talking with patients, a teaching approach.* Nuffield Provincial Hospitals Trust, London.

Weatherall D (1996) Keynote address presented to *Teaching about communication in medicine.* International Conference, St. Catherine's College, July 25, Oxford, England.

Weinberger M, Greene JY and Mamlin JJ (1981) The impact of clinical encounter events on patient and physician satisfaction. *Soc Sci Med.* **15E**: 239–44.

Werner A and Schneider JM (1974) Teaching medical students interactional skills: a research-based course in the doctor–patient relationship. *N Engl J Med.* **290**: 1232–7.

Westberg J and Jason H (1993) *Collaborative clinical education: the foundation of effective health care*. Springer, New York.

Westberg J and Jason H (1994) *Teaching creatively with video: fostering reflection, communication and other clinical skills*. Springer, New York.

Whitehouse CR (1991) The teaching of communication skills in United Kingdom medical schools. *Med Educ*. **25**: 311–18.

Whitehouse CR, Morris P and Marks B (1984) The role of actors in teaching communication. *Med Educ*. **18**: 262–8.

Wissow LS, Roter DL and Wilson MEH (1994) Pediatrician interview style and mothers' disclosure of psychosocial issues. *Pediatrics*. **93**: 289–95.

Workshop Planning Committee (1992) Consensus statement from the workshop on teaching and assessment of communication in Canadian medical schools. *Can Med Assoc J*. **147**: 1149–50.

World Federation for Medical Education (1994) Proceedings of the world summit on medical education. *Med Educ* **28** (Suppl. 1).

Zeeman EC (1976) Catastrophe theory. *Scientific American*. **April**: 65.

Appendix 1:
Sample communication
curricula

Appendix 1 presents two communication curricula that illustrate how to put the material in this book and its companion title into practice. The undergraduate and residency curricula presented here share the same broad objectives:

- to promote collaboration and partnership between physician and patient which will ensure accurate and efficient information exchange in a supportive climate
- to lay the foundations for developing communication skills to a professional level of competence
- to improve physician–patient communication *in practice*.

Overview of an undergraduate communication curriculum:
Faculty of Medicine, University of Calgary, Alberta, Canada

Co-Directors: CJ Heaton, MD and SM Kurtz, PhD

This book and its companion title describe the structures, principles, theory and research on which we have based the communication curriculum for medical students at the University of Calgary. Evolving over the past 20 years, Calgary's communication curriculum currently includes the following components:

- a three-phase, self-contained Communication Course
- a two-part Integrative Course

- two Medical Skills Evaluations
- the Family Medicine Clerkship and Evaluation.

Communication is also an overlaid and developing focus in medical students' courses on ethics; culture, health and illness; family violence; the well physician; and in other clerkships. Among other current initiatives, we are in the process of collaborating with the Human Development Course to create a more explicit emphasis on communicating with normal and challenged children and with adolescents and their families through both standardized patients and opportunities to interact with real patients and family members.

Resources

The resources identified in this section have also been assembled over many years. Initially a stand-alone course and later part of the Clinical Skills Course (which housed communication, physical examination and behavioural development), communication is now part of the *Medical Skills Program*. This combines into one administrative structure course, and evaluations on communication, physical examination, ethics, culture and gender related to health and illness, medical informatics and technology, well physician, evidence-based practice and the integrative courses. The program chairman and directors of these courses meet periodically for planning, discussion, updates and ongoing efforts at coordination of coursework and evaluations. This offers opportunities for integration and cooperation between these courses, all of which emphasize the development of clinical and personal skills. We also attempt to coordinate with the Clerkship, which comprises students' entire third year and provides supervised clinical experience in the various specialty areas. Dedicated time for the program is continuous throughout the first two years of the three year medical school curriculum.

The *Calgary–Cambridge observation guides* and their earlier versions have delineated the skills content and objectives of the curriculum, and provided focus and continuity since we began the program in 1977. In keeping with the helical model on which the curriculum is built, we use two separate guides which allow us to introduce the skills progressively at different points in the curriculum, rather than all together. Guide One focuses on the information-gathering interview and Guide Two on explanation and planning. The two-guide version we currently use is included in Appendix 2. We also supply a *medical history form*, a third 'guide' which simply lists and reminds students of the sections of the traditional medical history, i.e. the content of the information-gathering interview, and leaves space for observers and interviewers to record details as each part of the history is gathered.

The Guides are a primary resource which students and facilitators use repeatedly to help structure and focus practice, observation, feedback and discussion of personal experience and the literature. With the addition of satisfactory and unsatisfactory columns, the Guides are also used in certifying evaluations.

Other resources currently include the *Standardized Patient Program* (which originated with the Communication Course and now serves the broader faculty, including residency and CME programs), the *Volunteer Patient Data-base* (for communication and/or physical examination), and the *Medical Skills Centre*. Set up for small-group teaching and evaluation, the Centre is made up of double rooms equipped with one-way mirrors (examining room on one side, small-group seating and audio-video controls on the other), videotape equipment and computers. A collection of *print and video resource materials* for the communication curriculum is housed together in the *Bacs Medical Learning Resource Centre*, a self-learning area serving the Medical Skills Program and the Clerkship which includes print, video and computer resources, models and specimens and a radiology museum. And of course this book and its companion title are now the major texts, taking the place of the earlier Riccardi and Kurtz (1983) text.

The patients with whom students interact are:

- *real patients* from communication facilitators' practices, the volunteer patient data-base or the hospital adjacent to the medical school (all volunteer their time and portray themselves)
- *standardized patients* portrayed by professional actors from the community
- students or the co-directors who occasionally *role play* themselves with enough details changed to protect privacy.

All our standardized patient cases are based on real cases contributed over many years by faculty and community physicians. They range from cases presented in one or two pages which include history details and comments on personality, affect and specific communication challenges (e.g. for Phases 1 and 2) to more complex records which include additional findings on physical examination, laboratory and investigation reports, X-rays and MRIs, progression of events over time and possibly multiple visits (e.g. for the Integrative Course and the evaluations).

Leadership for the program comes from a family medicine doctor and a communication specialist, who co-direct the three phases of the self-contained Communication Course. Their roles include organizing the course and its materials, recruiting and training facilitators, developing standardized patient cases and overseeing recruitment of 'real' patients, evaluation and remedial work. The co-directors have also been integrally involved in initiating and implementing the Integrative Course, Medical Skills Evaluations, Medical Skills Program (including the Standardized Patient Program and the Medical Skills Centre) and Family Practice Clerkship. The director of the Standardized Patient Program is a professional actor/director/ producer who recruits, organizes, trains and follows up the standardized patients.

Small group facilitators (called 'preceptors' in Calgary) also play a major leadership role. They include 18 community and faculty physicians for the Communication Course mostly from family medicine with a few from psychiatry and sometimes other specialties – many have been with the course for over 15 years. Another 12 join for each of the Integrative Courses mostly from the specialties and some from family medicine. Additional doctors serve as preceptors in the clerkships or as medical skills examiners. One way we have promoted communication is through the involvement of this broad spectrum of faculty and community physicians. Newly recruited facilitators are often physicians who have been through earlier iterations of the curriculum as medical students at Calgary.

Others who influence the curriculum are the chair of the Medical Skills Program, directors of the other courses and clerkships where communication plays a role, and doctors who work with students in these courses.

Components of the communication curriculum

Table 1 presents the components of Calgary's communication curriculum in their chrono-logical order of appearance and includes the logistics of timing, format and methods. The brief descriptions which follow outline the primary focus of each component and our helical approach to improving communication skills, integrating them with other clinical skills and ensuring ongoing development of the curriculum. All components of the curriculum are mandatory and Calgary requires attendance at all sessions where patients (real or standard-ized) are present, i.e. all our small-group sessions.

PHASE 1 OF THE COMMUNICATION COURSE

This focuses on developing the skills of initiating interaction, gathering information and building relation-ship with patients (Guide One skills), in the context of taking a complete medical history (the medical history form). Skills of peer and self-assessment and working with colleagues are secondary focuses in all phases. Phase 1 begins with an orientation lecture which introduces the communication curriculum, including some of the research and theory behind it. Thereafter, all but one session are done in small groups. We randomly divide the 72 students per class into groups of four or five under the leadership of a preceptor who is a practising doctor; groups remain the same for Phases 1 and 2. While the learning group observes and makes notes, students take turns interviewing real patients who present current or ongoing problems for which they have recently needed medical attention and standardized patients who portray problems students are studying in systems courses which run concurrently with the Communication Course (fever, sore throat, a request for a periodic health examination, reticulo-endothelial and musculo-skeletal problems and a combination medical/ethics problem regarding boundaries between physician and patient). Occasionally, students or the co-directors volunteer to role play themselves as patients (changing some details of history to protect privacy). Both chronic and acute care are addressed. Here and in Phase 2 all interviews are videotaped for possible partial review during the session and full review during students' independent study time.

After each interview, the physician-led small group invites the patient to give feedback, discusses issues and problems which the interviewer (or the interview) raises, offers their own feedback to the interviewer (sometimes assisted by replaying sections of the videotape), tries out alternative approaches and discusses relevant experience, theory and research. Rather than attempting the complete history all at once, groups begin with initiation only, then add in history of present illness, past history, drug and allergy histories and other parts of the complete history in progressive fashion across the first six or eight weeks. Guide One skills can also be introduced progressively. At appropriate times students are directed to read each skills chapter of the companion book, i.e. the chapter on overall curriculum, initiation, gath-ering information, building relationship and closing. To enhance their participation and small-group skills, we also encourage them to look at Chapters 1 and 3–6 of this book. A few weeks into Phase 1, students participate in a large-group version of the first half of the Bayer Work-shop on Clinician–Patient Communication, focusing on skills of engagement and empathy. This introduces them to an alternative way to conceptualize communication with patients (Keller and Carrol 1994) which complements and reinforces the approach taken in the Guides. Physical examination and systems courses run concurrently with the Communication Course in the medical school's clinical presentation curriculum.

Table 1: Logistics

Components	When	Formats	Methods
Phase 1	1st year, Sept–Nov 12 wks × 2 hrs = 24 hrs	1 large-group lecture/discussion 1 large-group workshop (Bayer: Phys-Pt Comm Part 1) 10 small-group sessions Facilitators from family med, psychiatry and some specialties	**CCGuide One and Med hx form** Real patients Standardized patients – 13 cases Student role play Vtr of students' interviews (videotape recording)
Phase 2	1st year, April–May 4 wks × 2 hrs = 8 hrs	4 small-group sessions Facilitators groups as for Phase 1	**CCGuide One and Med hx form** Standardized patients – 9 cases Vtr of students' interviews
Medical Skills I Evaluation	1st year, May Exam: 1.5 hrs Tutorial: 1.5–2 hrs	Exam: student interviewing SPs Tutorial: 2 students and examiner do video review of skills	**CCGuide One and Med hx form** 4 OSCE Stations – 3 cases Standardized patients Vtr of students' interviews Paper and pencil Video review/tutorial
Integrative A	1st year, June 2 wks and 2 days (full-time)	Small-group sessions (# determined by group) Facilitators from family med and specialties	**CCGuide One** Standardized patients – 11 cases Vtr of student interviews
Phase 3	2nd year, Nov 2 wks × 2 hrs = 4 hrs Feb 3 wks × 2 hrs = 6 hrs	2 large-group workshop sessions (Bayer: Difficult Phys-Pt Rels) 1 large-group lecture/demo/disc 1 large-group workshop (Bayer: Phys-Pt Comm, Part 2) 2 student role play exercises	**CCGuides One and Two** Lecture/discussion and exercises Demo video tapes Student role play
Medical Skills II Evaluation	2nd year, Feb Exam: 3 hrs Tutorial: 1.5–2 hrs	Exam: student interviewing SPs Tutorial: 2 students and examiner	**CCGuide One and selected items of Guide Two** 6 OSCE Stations – 5 cases Standardized patients Vtr Paper and pencil Videotape review/tutorial
Integrative B	2nd year, April 2 wks and 2 days (full-time)	Small-group sessions Facilitators from family prac and specialties	**CCGuides One and Two** Standardized patients – 17 cases Vtr of student interviews
Family Practice Clerkship	3rd year, 4 weeks Comm components in clerkship and evaluation	Preceptor led, Family phys one on one	**CCGuides One and Two** 7 OSCE Stations Real patients Standardized patients (exam only) Vtr

Communication also receives attention in other Medical Skills Program courses – Culture, health and illness; Ethics; Family violence; other clerkship evaluations, e.g. ObGyn, Psychiatry and Surgery.

PHASE 2 OF THE COMMUNICATION COURSE

This reviews and refines the Phase 1 skills and adds the complexity of difficult physician–patient situations. We rely entirely on standardized patients in this phase. Portraying nine cases, the standardized patients permit us to present students with selected medical problems from a variety of systems and with specific communication issues, e.g. patients from another culture, unwanted pregnancy and communication challenges, e.g. patients who are in pain, angry or experiencing an emergency. Here we also begin to bring in how to give preliminary information to patients and how to make the connection between communication, clinical reasoning and problem solving. We follow the same pattern of practice, observation, feedback (assisted sometimes by replaying sections of the videotape), discussion and rehearsal of alternatives. Full videotape review occurs outside class time. We direct students to review the skills material from Phase 1, to read Chapter 7 of the companion book and to revisit Chapter 6 of this book, this time applying it to working with and educating patients. An extensive bibliography of materials available in the Learning Centre is provided.

MEDICAL SKILLS I EVALUATION

This assesses communication skills emphasized in Phases 1 and 2 and offers a first opportunity to integrate these skills with physical examination, knowledge from the systems courses and clinical presentation problems, interpretation of data and problem solving and, most recently, ethical and cultural issues (which are built into some standardized patient cases). The Medical Skills Evaluations serve three purposes: certifying evaluation, integration, and teaching and learning (including review and reinforcement). Communication skills are examined primarily in Stations 1-A and 1-B, which relate to a single case (the other stations assess other parts of the Medical Skills Program). In 1-A students take a 25-minute complete history from a standardized patient who is new to them. This interview is videotaped. Given a few minutes to organize notes and thoughts, students progress to 1-B (up to 45 minutes) where they present the history to an examiner, present a problem list and tentative hypotheses and describe what they would do on physical examination. Examiners correct errors and fill in missing information regarding the history and then ask students to perform specific aspects of the physical examination. Next, the correct physical findings and results of investigation are given to students who are asked to interpret the results and then to 'update' their problem list and discuss their different diagnosis. Standardized patients and physician examiners evaluate three stations during the exam itself (Stations 1-B, 2 and 3) using detailed check-lists and worksheets. The history-taking interview in Station 1-A is assessed after the examination itself during a mandatory video review and tutorial. Students sign up in pairs with a Communication Course preceptor/examiner (different from their small-group facilitator) to observe, discuss and evaluate each student's communication skills from the videotaped interview. To enhance discussions of how communication process skills affect the quality of the information gathered or the student's clinical reasoning processes or interpretation of physical examination, students bring to the tutorial the paperwork their Station 1-B evaluator completed during the exam (i.e. evaluation and feedback sheets regarding details of student performance from the presentation of the history, physical examination of the patient, interpretation of data and problem solving) and the standardized patient's written check-list and comments.

All three participants in the tutorial watch the videotapes to identify communication weaknesses and strengths, work on problem areas and refinement of skills, rehearse alternatives, fill in the evaluation forms (including their own performances) and conclude with a recommendation of satisfactory or unsatisfactory for the station and suggestions for 'next steps'. An evaluation committee reviews results. The evaluation is certifying, i.e. throughout Calgary's mastery learning medical program, students must obtain a satisfactory mark or do remedial work and retake the examination successfully before they can move on. We intentionally place the two Medical Skills Evaluations some weeks after the components which precede them in order to provide timely opportunity for further review and reinforcement of communication skills. We coordinate the Medical Skills and Family Medicine Clerkship evaluations in order to assess progressively medical skills and their integration with knowledge base and the other clinical skills.

INTEGRATIVE COURSE A

This focuses on integrating the clinical skills of communication, physical examination and problem solving with medical technical knowledge students have gained to this point in their training and on deepening their understanding, skill and professional behaviour in all those areas. This course gives students opportunity to review and enhance their Guide One communication and other clinical skills in the context of standardized patients, to work on weaknesses identified during their Medical Skills Evaluation and to make connections between communications, physical examination and problem solving.

As described more fully in Chapter 8, students practise with up to 11 standardized patients who portray an array of specific medical problems and psycho-social issues and introduce a variety of communication issues and challenges, e.g. culture, gender, multi-party interviewing, age, death and dying, bereavement. Standardized cases include chronic and acute care as well as opportunities for communicating with patients over time during multiple visits. Small groups of six to eight students under the guidance of a preceptor (who is a physician) divide the patient contact for any given case. For example, the group observes as one student takes the history and performs the physical examination, a second student offers preliminary counselling (explanation of preliminary findings, lab tests, diagnostic procedures), a third does definitive counselling (explanation, planning and decision making) and a fourth the follow-up visit. After each interaction with the patient and often with the patient as a participant, the group gives feedback on skills, discusses clinical reasoning, explores issues and challenges, discusses and tries out alternative approaches, plans 'next steps', identifies and corrects knowledge gaps and learning issues, works with resource people in the community, etc. All of this typically takes place over a time period of two to five days for each case.

PHASE 3 OF THE COMMUNICATION COURSE

This reviews Phase 1 and 2 skills and introduces communication skills, principles and research associated with information giving, explanation and planning, and shared decision making (CC Guide Two). It also emphasizes the skills of giving bad news and working with difficult physician–patient relationships. Phase 3 in November consists of the Bayer Workshop on Difficult Relationships, which combines videotape depicting potential difficult relationships with lecture, slides, discussion and exercises and is presented in large-group format. Phase 3 continues in February with lecture, discussion and the presentation of a videotape which demonstrates the skills of disclosing bad news about cancer to several different patients (Brod *et al*. 1986). Students then try out some of these skills by participating in an exercise in which some of them volunteer to learn and play the role of a specific patient (thus giving them an opportunity to see things from the patient's perspective), while other students volunteer to conduct the explanation and planning consultation or observe and provide feedback. Finally, students participate in the second half of the Bayer Workshop on Clinician–Patient Communication, focusing on skills of enlistment and education. We direct them to read the chapter on explanation and planning in our companion book and to review the other skills material, including Chapter 6 of this book.

MEDICAL SKILLS II EVALUATION

This follows the same objectives and pattern as Medical Skills I, including review of skills previously learned – one two-part 'long' station (as for Station 1-A and B above) and three shorter stations in which students take focused histories, undertake relevant physical examination and discuss appropriate information regarding differential diagnosis and 'next steps' with patients. In recent years short cases also assessed communication skills associated with ethics, cultural issues and the well physician. Once again this evaluation, and the video review and tutorial that are part of it, sets students up for the next component where exploring explanation and planning skills in greater depth becomes a major objective. While higher levels of skill are anticipated, many students find that their skills are beginning to atrophy from lack of focused attention and practice, so the review aspect of this evaluation takes on particular importance.

INTEGRATIVE COURSE B

This follows the same pattern as Integrative A, but here emphasis regarding communication is given to patient management and experimenting with and developing the skills on Guide Two. Some cases are more complex than for Integrative A and more demanding multi-systems problems are included. This course immediately precedes the beginning of clerkship so all the systems courses and their clinical presentation cases have been completed by this point.

FAMILY PRACTICE CLERKSHIP

This offers students opportunities for observation and supervised practice with real patients in community and staff physicians' practices. The seven-station OSCE evaluation for this clerkship assesses skills on both Guides One and Two, with an emphasis on integration and on demonstration of explanation and planning skills and negotiation regarding 'next steps' in investigation and management. The evaluation features three focused stations and one case which involves four stations: focused history and relationship building, relevant physical exam and discussing plans with the patient for further investigations, write-up of the medical record or presentation of the case to a preceptor, and a repeat visit with the patient two weeks 'later' to determine events since the last visit and discuss results of investigations and 'next steps'. Again, all interviews are videotaped. Feedback is given via written sheets on each station and small-group discussion with each other, facilitators, rotation directors, and standardized patients about clinical problems and the clerk's performance. Students review videos of physician–patient interactions from each of the evaluation's stations, this time with an emphasis on self-evaluation (using the formal evaluation sheets) and ideally preceptor and peer feedback.

One other part of Calgary's communication curriculum is integration or coordination between communication and other courses in the Medical Skills Program or other clerkships. Examples of this less structured aspect of the curriculum are presented in Chapter 8.

Overview of a communication curriculum for residency: The Vocational Training Scheme for General Practice, Cambridge, England

J Draper, FRCGP and JD Silverman, FRCGP

The communication skills curriculum for residency training that we describe here has been gradually developed over the last six years as an integral and increasingly important component of the general practice residency training programme in Cambridge, England. It has become the blueprint for communication curricula in general practice training throughout the Anglian region.

The structure of residency training for general practice in England, known as 'vocational training', is as follows:

- a three-year training programme
  - two years rotation through hospital-based specialist attachments
  - a one-year community-based general practice training attachment to specific accredited training practices
- weekly day release from training practice to attend small-group teaching sessions
- two groups of teachers
  - trainers (community-based general practitioners) who teach one-to-one in individual training practices
  - course organizers (general practitioners with a part-time educational post) who are responsible for organizing and facilitating the day release small-group teaching sessions.

The communication curriculum occurs within the weekly day release programme that runs throughout the general practice-based year of vocational training. Many issues compete for limited teaching time within the day release course: clinical knowledge, patient management, attitudinal group work, practice organization, practical skills such as minor surgery and child health surveillance, project work and audits all vie for the available time. The communication programme that we describe here therefore represents a compromise – although it has been a major development in communication skills training within the region, it should be seen as a basic minimum rather than a position of excellence.

Our approach to structuring the communication curriculum in residency training combines three types of experiential learning:

1 *Opportunistic video work on real cases.* Vocational training in British general practice has embraced the medium of video recording for many years and the submission of a selection

of residents' videotaped consultations with real patients is now an obligatory part of summative assessment for entry into the specialty of general practice. Almost all training practices have their own video equipment and residents can therefore readily videotape their own consultations for educational purposes. Residents can bring examples of difficult consultations which enables a real life problem-based approach to communication skills teaching to be taken. In Chapter 5, we discussed how to run such opportunistic video sessions and how to use the Calgary–Cambridge guide as an aid to observation and feedback.

2 *Planned work on sections of the interview.* Once opportunistic work on individual cases is underway, it is possible to introduce other ways of working. Along with sessions about problem cases, we can intersperse sessions exploring the problems that occur in each section of the interview (beginning the consultation, information gathering, relationship building, explanation and planning, ending). We use videotapes of residents' real consultations or simulated cases to obtain an understanding of the skills that are important in each phase of the consultation. This enables learners to consider objectives and to identify, observe and rehearse basic skills. As the curriculum proceeds, each of the five sections of the consultation can be explored sequentially; this process serves to reinforce and structure the learning from opportunistic sessions.

3 *Planned work on specific communication issues.* A third kind of experiential work uses simulated patients or trigger tapes to introduce communication issues that might well not arise during opportunistic work on real video material. If we rely entirely on videos of real cases it is difficult to ensure, for instance, that examples of breaking bad news or cultural issues or addiction will surface. Planned sessions using simulated patient roles or trigger tapes can be interspersed with the above two formats to enable further skills work relevant to specific issues to be undertaken.

The communication curriculum described requires a total of two days of teaching within each 12-week term. The sessions are held in both the medical postgraduate centre attached to Addenbrooke's teaching hospital in Cambridge and also, for at least one whole day session per term, in the more pleasant teaching environment of a country house some distance from the city and away from potential interruptions. The day release course offers many opportunities that are not possible within each individual training practice:

• peer assessment, learning and support
• small-group work, with a ratio of one facilitator to six residents
• greater exchange of approaches
• easier availability of rehearsal through role play
• simulated patients
• an ongoing planned curriculum structured throughout the year
• skilled group facilitators
• facilitators who are knowledgeable about the theory and research concerning communication in medicine.

Overlays within the vocational training scheme

Course organizers also take every opportunity to bring out the communication challenges in clinical problems covered in other parts of the day release course. When hormone replacement therapy is discussed, we examine not only the knowledge and problem solving required to be an effective doctor in general practice, but also explore and preferably role play the difficulties of negotiating a course of action for an individual patient, the intricacies of discovering the patient's perspective of her needs and the problems of explaining relative risk. It is not just knowing information but applying that knowledge in action that is important. When psychosexual problems are discussed, it is not only the details of what is available to a man with premature ejaculation that need to be highlighted, but also the communication challenge of discussing such sensitive and embarrassing issues and knowing what language to use with the patient. 'Overlaying' communication issues throughout the course reinforces the more formal work performed in the communication curriculum *per se*.

Teaching within the individual training practices

Although the day release programme establishes a strong foundation for developing communication skills, it provides insufficient time to give ongoing personal attention to each resident. As the programme progresses through the year, it is necessary to reinforce and complement the learners' day release experience. Trainers continue to give one-to-one communication skills teaching via opportunistic videos in the parent practices. Regular one-to-one consultation skills teaching in training practices validates the importance of this subject to residents and enables frequent experience of videoing, observation and feedback. This one-to-one teaching works hand-in-hand with the expert groupwork teaching of the structured communication curriculum presented during the day release scheme. All trainers therefore require training themselves in communication skills teaching and this is an ongoing responsibility of course organizers (*see* Chapter 9).

Both one-to-one teaching and overlays of communication contribute significantly to the helical process of reiteration, review and refinement of skills that is required for doctors to put learning into practice.

Term 1

Two to three-hour session

INTRODUCTION TO COMMUNICATION SKILLS TEACHING – WHY, WHAT AND HOW

A combination of exercises, mini-lectures and demonstrations via trigger tapes and facilitators' video recordings of their own consultations covering:

- possible gains and concerns of looking at communication skills
- why teach communication skills (*based on material in Chapter 1*)
- the importance of structure and skills
- explaining the Calgary–Cambridge guide (*based on Chapter 2*)
- why look at your own videos and not just prepared tapes: the importance of observation, rehearsal and feedback (*based on Chapter 3*)
- modelling agenda-led outcome-based feedback and descriptive feedback by looking at a facilitator's tape (*see Chapter 5*).

Whole day

Three two-hour sessions exploring:

1 opportunistic video work
2 planned section: initiating the consultation.

SESSIONS ONE AND TWO

- Getting started: developing a supportive environment and setting agendas (*see Chapter 6*).
- Opportunistic video sessions using residents' videotaped real consultations.

SESSION THREE

- Initiating the consultation: using residents' own tapes to explore objectives and skills in this section of the consultation.

ENDING

- Feedback about what was learned, methodology, supportiveness and value of session.
- Summary of learning – tying into the guides, developing a conceptual framework.
- How to further progress learning by practising in the consulting room and by continuing video work with trainers in individual training practices

Two-hour session

A SPECIFIC COMMUNICATION ISSUE IN GENERAL PRACTICE

- Choose an issue that fits in with the clinical content of a session to be explored within the day release programme, e.g. drug therapy in depression, asthma, child developmental assessment, hormone replacement therapy, death and dying.
- Attach a specific communication issue that you or the group wish to explore to one of these subject areas, e.g. child developmental assessment – discovering postnatal depression in mother at six-week check.
- Develop simulated patient role prior to the session.
- Follow a traditional session on the clinical subject area with a two-hour session using role play with actor, then feedback and analysis discussing both issues of clinical content and specific communication challenges (content and process).
- Summarize the *core* and *issue-specific* skills and how they interrelate (*see Chapter 7 and companion book Chapter 7*).

Term 2

Whole day

Three two-hour sessions:

1 planned section: gathering information
2 opportunistic video work
3 specific communication issue: cultural.

SESSIONS ONE AND TWO

- Introductions, objectives, re-establish learning agendas.
- Exercise: objectives of the gathering information section of the consultations.
- Mini-lecture: introduction to gathering information, the link between communication skills and diagnostic hypothesis making, the disease–illness model.
- Opportunistic videos with specific reference to gathering information.

SESSION THREE

- Specific communication issue: cultural issues.
- Working with simulated patient to demonstrate the particular importance of the disease–illness model in differing cultural situations.

ENDING

- Feedback of what was learned, methodology, supportiveness and value of session.
- Summary of learning – tying into the guides, developing a conceptual framework.

Whole day

Three two-hour sessions:

1 planned section: building the relationship
2 opportunistic video work.

SESSIONS ONE AND TWO

- Introductions, objectives, re-establish learning agendas.
- Exercise: difficulties in relationship building with patients and patient groups that learners find difficult or awkward.
- Opportunistic videowork with specific reference to building the relationship: ask participants to bring videos of difficult consultations where they don't like or don't understand the patient, where they feel no rapport, etc.
- Teaching reempathy, acceptance and non-verbal communication – exercise in reverse role play, sinking yourself into the patient's shoes.

SESSION THREE

- Simulated patient scenario for relationship-building skills, e.g. a patient who breaks down in tears over marital violence where the doctor has little to offer except support, or a young patient, reluctant to talk, who admits being gay and cannot face telling parents.

Term 3

Whole day

Three two-hour sessions:

1 planned section: explanation and planning
2 opportunistic video work
3 specific communication issue: explanation of risk, confrontation.

SESSIONS ONE AND TWO

- Introductions, objectives, re-establish learning agendas.
- Mini-lecture: introduction to explanation and planning – evidence regarding problems, compliance and outcome (*see Chapter 1*).
- Opportunistic videos with specific reference if possible to explanation and planning.

SESSION THREE

- Specific communication issue: explanation of risk, confrontation.
- Working with simulated patient to demonstrate issues in explanation and planning and in particular explanation of risk and confrontation, e.g. patient who smokes, found to have

high blood pressure by practice nurse and asked to make appointment to see doctor, or a patient requesting hormone replacement therapy.

ENDING

- Feedback of what was learned, methodology, supportiveness, value of session.
- Summary of learning – tying into the guides, developing a conceptual framework.

Half day

One three-hour session – specific communication issue: breaking bad news

- Session on breaking bad news, using participant role play of 60-year-old man returning to GP for results of test that show carcinoma of oesophagus, or a woman with polyarthritis who returns for the results of tests which show that she has rheumatoid arthritis.

Half day

TWO TWO-HOUR SESSIONS – PULLING IT ALL TOGETHER/ENDING
Discussion of the structure and skills of a whole consultation.

SESSION ONE

- Opportunistic videos – looking at ending the consultation if possible (*see Chapter 6 of companion book*).

SESSION TWO

- Opportunistic videos – pulling together all the skills in the consultation, looking at the 'flow' of the consultation, individual style and behaviours.

ENDING THE CURRICULUM

- Feelings about communication now.
- Feedback on course.
- Where next?

Appendix 2:
The two-guide format of the *Calgary–Cambridge Observation Guide*

Calgary–Cambridge Observation Guide One – Interviewing The Patient

Student Name _____   Date _____

Initiating the session	Comments
1 GREETS patient and obtains patient's name 2 INTRODUCES SELF and clarifies role 3 DEMONSTRATES interest and RESPECT, attends to physical comfort (here and throughout interview) 4 IDENTIFIES AND CONFIRMS PATIENT'S PROBLEM LIST or issues, e.g. 'So headache, fever – anything else you'd like to talk about?' 5 NEGOTIATES AGENDA taking both patient's and doctor's perspective into account	
Gathering information *EXPLORATION OF PROBLEMS* 6 ENCOURAGES PATIENT TO TELL STORY of problem(s) from when first started to the present in own words (clarifies reason for presenting now) 7 Uses open and closed questioning techniques. APPROPRIATELY MOVES FROM OPEN TO CLOSED 8 LISTENS ATTENTIVELY, allows patient to complete statements without interruption and leaves space for patient to think before answering or go on after pausing 9 FACILITATES PATIENT'S RESPONSES VERBALLY AND NON-VERBALLY (use of encouragement, silence, repetition, paraphrasing, interpretation) 10 USES concise, EASILY UNDERSTOOD QUESTIONS AND COMMENTS, avoids or adequately explains jargon 11 CLARIFIES PATIENT'S STATEMENTS which are vague or need amplification, e.g. 'Could you explain what you mean by lightheaded' 12 ESTABLISHES DATES	

UNDERSTANDING THE PATIENT'S PERSPECTIVE

13 DETERMINES AND ACKNOWLEDGES PATIENT'S IDEAS,
   i.e. beliefs regarding cause
14 EXPLORES CONCERNS (including worries, effects
   on lifestyle) regarding each problem
15 DETERMINES PATIENT'S EXPECTATIONS
   regarding each problem
16 ENCOURAGES EXPRESSION OF FEELINGS AND
   THOUGHTS
17 PICKS UP VERBAL AND NON-VERBAL CLUES, i.e.
   body language, speech, facial expression, affect,
   CHECKS OUT and acknowledges as appropriate

STRUCTURING THE CONSULTATION

18 SUMMARIZES AT END OF A SPECIFIC LINE OF INQUIRY
   (present Hx, past Hx) to verify own interpretation
   of what patient has said, to ensure no important
   data were omitted
19 PROGRESSES from one section to another USING
   TRANSITIONAL STATEMENTS; includes rationale
   for next section
20 STRUCTURES interview in LOGICAL SEQUENCE
21 ATTENDS TO TIMING and keeping interview on task

Building relationship – facilitating patient's involvement

22 DEMONSTRATES APPROPRIATE NON-VERBAL BEHAVIOUR,
   e.g. eye contact, posture and position, movement,
   facial expression, use of voice
23 If READS, WRITES notes or uses computer,
   does IN A MANNER THAT DOES NOT INTERFERE
   WITH DIALOGUE OR RAPPORT
24 ACCEPTS LEGITIMACY OF PATIENT'S VIEWS; is
   not judgemental
25 EMPATHIZES WITH AND SUPPORTS PATIENT,
   e.g. expresses concern, understanding,
   willingness to help, acknowledges coping efforts
   and appropriate self-care
26 DEALS SENSITIVELY WITH EMBARRASSING AND
   DISTURBING TOPICS and physical pain
27 APPEARS CONFIDENT AND reasonably relaxed
28 SHARES THINKING with patient WHEN APPROPRIATE
   to encourage patient's involvement, e.g.
   'What I'm thinking now is ...'

Explaining and planning – closing the session

29 GIVES EXPLANATION AT APPROPRIATE TIMES (avoids giving advice, information, opinions prematurely)

30 GIVES INFORMATION IN CLEAR, WELL-ORGANIZED, complete fashion without overloading patient; avoids or explains jargon

31 CHECKS PATIENT'S UNDERSTANDING AND ACCEPTANCE of explanation and plans; ensures that concerns have been addressed

32 ENCOURAGES PATIENT TO DISCUSS ANY ADDITIONAL POINTS and provides him/her with opportunity to do so, e.g. 'Are there any questions you'd like to ask or anything at all you'd like to discuss further?'

33 CLOSES INTERVIEW BY SUMMARIZING briefly, CONTRACTING WITH PATIENT REGARDING NEXT STEPS for patient and physician

Calgary–Cambridge Observation Guide Two – Explanation and Planning

Student Name _____   Date _____

Explanation and planning	Comments
PROVIDING THE CORRECT AMOUNT AND TYPE OF INFORMATION 1 INITIATES: summarizes to date, determines expectations, sets agenda 2 ASSESSES PATIENT'S STARTING POINT: asks for patient's prior knowledge early, discovers extent of patient's wish for information 3 CHUNKS AND CHECKS: gives information in assimilable chunks, checks for understanding, uses patient's response as a guide to how to proceed 4 ASKS patient WHAT OTHER INFORMATION WOULD BE HELPFUL, e.g. aetiology, prognosis 5 GIVES EXPLANATION AT APPROPRIATE TIMES: avoids giving advice, information or reassurance prematurely	
AIDING ACCURATE RECALL AND UNDERSTANDING 6 ORGANIZES EXPLANATION: divides into discrete sections, develops a logical sequence 7 USES EXPLICIT CATEGORIZATION OR SIGNPOSTING, e.g. 'There are three important things that I would like to discuss. First ... now shall we move on to ...' 8 USES REPETITION AND SUMMARIZING: to reinforce information 9 LANGUAGE: uses concise, easily understood statements, avoids or explains jargon 10 USES VISUAL METHODS OF CONVEYING INFORMATION: diagrams, models, written information and instructions 11 CHECKS PATIENT'S UNDERSTANDING OF INFORMATION GIVEN (or plans made), e.g. by asking patient to restate in own words; clarifies as necessary	

INCORPORATING THE PATIENT'S PERSPECTIVE –
ACHIEVING SHARED UNDERSTANDING

12 RELATES EXPLANATIONS TO PATIENT'S ILLNESS
FRAMEWORK: to previously elicited beliefs,
concerns and expectations
13 PROVIDES OPPORTUNITIES/ENCOURAGES PATIENT TO
CONTRIBUTE: to ask questions, seek clarification or
express doubts: responds appropriately
14 PICKS UP VERBAL AND NON-VERBAL CUES, e.g.
patient's need to contribute information or ask
questions, information overload, distress
15 ELICITS PATIENT'S BELIEFS, REACTIONS AND FEELINGS
regarding information given, decisions, terms
used; acknowledges and addresses where
necessary

PLANNING – SHARED DECISION MAKING

16 SHARES OWN THOUGHTS: ideas, thought processes
and dilemmas
17 INVOLVES PATIENT by making suggestions rather
than directives
18 ENCOURAGES PATIENT TO CONTRIBUTE
their IDEAS, suggestions, preferences,
beliefs
19 NEGOTIATES A MUTUALLY ACCEPTABLE PLAN
20 OFFERS CHOICES: encourages patient to make
choices and decisions to level they wish
21 CHECKS WITH PATIENT: if accepts plans, if
concerns have been addressed

Options in explanation and planning

IF DISCUSSING OPINION AND SIGNIFICANCE
OF PROBLEM

22 OFFERS OPINION of what is going on and names
if possible
23 REVEALS RATIONALE for opinion
24 EXPLAINS causation, seriousness, expected
outcome, short and long-term consequences
25 CHECKS PATIENT'S UNDERSTANDING of what has
been said
26 ELICITS PATIENT'S BELIEFS, REACTIONS AND CONCERNS,
e.g. if opinion matches patient's thoughts,
acceptability, feelings

IF NEGOTIATING MUTUAL PLAN OF ACTION

27 DISCUSSES OPTIONS, e.g. no action, investigation, medication or surgery, non-drug treatments (physiotherapy, walking aids, fluids, counselling), preventative measures

28 PROVIDES INFORMATION on action or treatment offered:
   (a) name
   (b) steps involved, how it works
   (c) benefits and advantages
   (d) possible side-effects

29 ELICITS PATIENT'S UNDERSTANDING, REACTIONS AND CONCERNS about plans and treatments, including acceptability

30 OBTAINS PATIENT'S VIEW of NEED for action, PERCEIVED BENEFITS, BARRIERS, MOTIVATION; accepts and advocates alternative viewpoint as necessary

31 TAKES PATIENT'S LIFESTYLE, BELIEFS, cultural BACKGROUND and ABILITIES INTO CONSIDERATION

32 ENCOURAGES PATIENT to be involved in implementing plans, TO TAKE RESPONSIBILITY and be self-reliant

33 ASKS ABOUT PATIENT SUPPORT SYSTEMS, discusses other support available

IF DISCUSSING INVESTIGATIONS AND PROCEDURES

34 PROVIDES CLEAR INFORMATION ON PROCEDURES including what patient might experience and how patient will be informed of results

35 RELATES PROCEDURES TO TREATMENT PLAN: value and purpose

36 ENCOURAGES QUESTIONS AND EXPRESSION OF THOUGHTS regarding potential anxieties or negative outcome

Closing the session

37 SUMMARIZES session briefly

38 CONTRACTS WITH PATIENT regarding next steps for patient and physician

39 SAFETY NETS APPROPRIATELY and explains possible unexpected outcomes. What to do if plan is not working, when and how to seek help

40 CHECK THAT PATIENT AGREES and is comfortable with plan and ASKS IF ANY CORRECTION, QUESTIONS or other items to discuss

Index

Author Index